MW01028133

Minute Health Tips

---

*Medical Advice and
Facts at a Glance*

Thomas G. Welch, M.D.

Minute Health Tips: Medical Advice and Facts at a Glance © 1991 by Thomas G. Welch, M.D.

Library of Congress Cataloging-in-Publication Data

Welch, Thomas G., M.D.
      Minute health tips: medical advice and facts at a
          glance/Thomas G. Welch, M.D.
              p.   cm.
      Includes bibliographical references and index.
      ISBN 0-937721-85-9 $8.95
      1. Medicine, Popular--Encyclopedias. I. Title
      RC81.A2W45   1991
      610--dc20   91-27960
                                                   CIP

Edited by: Carol Frick, Donna Hoel
Cover Design: Eric Lecy
Text Design/Production Manager: Nancy Nies
Printed in the United States of America

10 9 8 7 6 5 4 3 2 1

Published by: DCI/CHRONIMED Publishing
P.O. Box 47945
Minneapolis, MN 55447-9727

Dedication

This book is dedicated to the memory of my father,
Dr. Harold V. Welch.

This book is not meant to replace your physician. Rather, these health tips are intended to provide guidelines and information that might indicate a visit to your doctor is necessary.

With grateful acknowledgement to WTVG, Channel 13, Toledo, Ohio, for the opportunity to use the medium of television to inform the public about medical issues.

With further acknowledgement to St. Vincent Medical Center, Toledo, Ohio, for assistance in presenting these health tips.

I gratefully acknowledge the technical assistance of my office staff, as well as the understanding of my medical partners: Pooran C. Barman, M.D., Jeffrey C. Maludy, M.D., and Elizabeth Attig, M.D.

TABLE OF CONTENTS

How This Book Came About

Several years ago, our local NBC outlet put out an urgent call for a Valentine's Day commentary on heart problems for the 6 o'clock news. Dr. Thomas Welch agreed to tackle the last-minute challenge.

Professional-looking in his trademark gray lab coat, Dr. Tom—as his friends have dubbed him—faced the cameras. Despite having been honed in a medical training system that appears to revel in the art of obfuscation, Dr. Tom sailed through the one-minute slot in crisp, clear, and concise style.

Buoyed by positive reviews and the public's desire for accurate and timely health news, TV-13 soon made Dr. Tom a Monday night program feature.

Over the years, Dr. Welch held constant to his formula for communication success: concise, practical medical tips to help the health-conscious consumer use medical care wisely and frugally—each topic covered within the 60-second limit of the television producer.

From how to avoid travelers' diarrhea to the benefits of an apple a day and the miracles of Mom's chicken soup, Dr. Tom captivated Toledo TV viewers.

These tips have been slightly edited to bring them up to current health information standards.

They are intended to be brief but sensible tips to help you become better informed and able to help yourself maintain good health and use professional medical care wisely and effectively.

Edward J. Pike, M.D., M.B.A.
Associate Vice President
Medical Education
St. Vincent Medical Center
Toledo, Ohio

FOREWORD

Americans today are not only making changes toward healthier lifestyles, they are also increasingly interested in making decisions about and participating in their own health care. There is clearly a "take charge" attitude by the public to manage its health.

Dr. Welch, first through his weekly television presentations highlighting health information, and now with these *Minute Health Tips*, pays heed to these desires of the health-conscious public. In a short, easy-to-read format, he addresses everyday health questions that might otherwise go unanswered. His health tips are not intended to be definitive essays on health issues, but they will certainly give his readers insight into health problems, offer comfort, and suggest approaches for resolving medical questions.

Dennis P. LeGolvan, M.D
St. Vincent Medical Center
Toledo, Ohio.

PREFACE

In 1984, I was asked by WTVG, Channel 13 in Toledo, Ohio (an NBC affiliate) to do occasional commentaries on heart disease and other medical topics. As the frequency of the appearances increased, I suggested that the television station commit to a particular day of the week for a health tip segment during the 6 o'clock news; they did it on a trial basis and I continued to provide a weekly health tip for about six years.

As time went on, I received more and more feedback from the viewing audience on the usefulness of these tips. I developed a greater appreciation for people's desire and need for relevant health information. It became apparent to me that misinformation, uncertainty, and fear in regard to medical issues were rampant among the general public. I found that people were anxious to participate in their own health care but simply didn't know how and didn't want to visit their doctor just to ask routine health advice. I also found that explaining symptoms and diseases in simple and easy-to-understand terms relieved a lot of anxiety. Although one minute was not sufficient to cover a particular topic in depth, it was adequate to provide guidelines to determine if and when a person needed to seek medical attention.

It is vitally important for people to participate in their own health care on an informed basis. Having correct medical information not only helps with disease prevention, it also makes doctor visits more useful and informative; the more that a patient understands about a particular disease process, the better questions can be asked of the physician.

But how many weighty and encyclopedic lay medical texts gather dust on the shelf? I believe there is a need for a convenient and readable guide to everyday medical questions and problems. Because of my involvement and interest in informing the public about medical issues, I decided to compile what I felt were some of the more prevalent medical problems of the 1990s and put them in an easy-to-read format that would not take more than a minute or two to cover. These tips are not intended to be an exhaustive analysis of these medical problems, but simply useful guidelines.

I hope this book will inform you, will allay some anxiety in regard to medical problems, and will help you participate in your own health care in a meaningful and understanding way.

Thomas G. Welch, M.D.

CIRCULATION AND INNER EAR PROBLEMS

Growing numbers of us routinely take to the air on business and pleasure trips. Occasionally, we might encounter some flight-related discomforts, especially when traveling long distances.

Prolonged sitting in an airplane seat may result in swelling of the feet, and can even lead to blood clots in the lower leg. This is caused by poor circulation due to inactivity and lack of muscle movement. It can affect people of all ages, even those in good health. If you are going on a long flight, try this: Flex your toes upward and hold for a count of 10, then put them down. Do this about eight times every 30 minutes. This will improve muscle activity and circulation. Of course, getting up and walking around will also help.

As the plane ascends or descends, changes in cabin pressure can cause the ears to plug. Swallowing helps to open up the tube in the inner ear where the pressure builds up. Chewing gum or sucking candy will encourage more frequent swallowing. Yawning is an even better activator of the muscle inside the head that opens up the drainage tube to unblock the ears. If this doesn't work, there is another method: Pinch your nostrils, take a mouthful of air, close your mouth, and then gently blow out, forcing the air into your pinched nose. Once you hear a loud pop, your ears will clear.

If you have a stuffy nose prior to boarding, using a decongestant or nasal spray an hour before take-off and an hour before landing will shrink the membranes in the nose that connect with the ears, allowing the ears to release the pressure (pop) more easily. If you have a bad cold, it would be wise to postpone your trip if possible. A plugged ear that will not unblock is painful and might require a trip to an emergency room at your destination.

ALLERGY TO EXERCISE

"RUNNING HIVES" AND ASTHMA

Many of us find exercising difficult, but did you know that there are people who are actually allergic to exercise?

They experience symptoms of itching, hives, wheezing, and abdominal cramping. The symptoms occur either several minutes after starting exercise or after the exercise is completed. These reactions usually subside spontaneously in 30 minutes to four hours. The reaction does not necessarily occur with each episode of exercise. Allergy to exercise is more commonly found in people who have other allergies (hay fever, etc.). Often, people who have only mild allergies to other things will find that exercise aggravates their reaction to those things even with minimum exposure to them. For instance, hay fever symptoms may be worse if you run during ragweed season. In addition, taking some medications, especially aspirin, before running can bring on this type of allergic reaction.

These are measures that can help prevent exercise-induced allergic reactions:
1. Take antihistamines or use an inhaled bronchodilator before exercise.
2. Avoiding eating for two hours or more before exercise.

As a precaution against a severe allergic reaction, you may want to have an adrenaline kit available, similar to that used for people who are allergic to bee stings.

If you have an allergy to exercise, a trial and error approach might be necessary, using both a combination of antihistamines and modification of your exercise routine. Your physician or allergist can help you explore remedies. Also, it's wise to exercise with a friend—so if you do have trouble you also have help.

HOW TO AVOID IRON DEFICIENCY

Anemia is a lack of red blood cells and is usually due to bleeding. Anemia is unusual in males, unless there is some hidden source of bleeding, such as the gastrointestinal tract (for example, ulcers or polyps). However, it is quite common in women who are still menstruating, especially if this monthly blood loss is not accompanied by adequate iron in the diet. Regardless of the cause of the anemia, it should always be investigated by your doctor.

Iron deficiency appears to be on the rise, perhaps because many people are avoiding red meat in their effort to cut cholesterol. However, red meat is one of the highest sources of iron! It's not easy to obtain large amounts of iron from the diet since only about 10 percent of dietary iron is absorbed from plant food and only about 40 percent from meats.

In order to ensure that adequate iron is being absorbed from your diet, include foods that have a high vitamin C content; vitamin C enhances the absorbability of iron. Preparing food in cast iron cookware can increase iron content up to threefold. Eat breads, cereals, and pastas that have been iron-fortified; the label on the package will tell you whether this has been done. Avoid drinking coffee or tea with your meals, since these beverages reduce iron absorption by as much as 50 percent. Finally, a glass of red wine with your meal can boost absorption of iron by as much as 300 percent.

AN APPLE A DAY

DOES IT REALLY KEEP THE DOCTOR AWAY?

You have heard that "an apple a day keeps the doctor away." This old saying turns out to have some truth to it. Consider this:

- A medium-sized apple contains only 80 calories, so it makes a nice, low-calorie snack.
- The crispness of it helps to keep your teeth clean.
- Apples contain vitamin A, good for your skin.
- Apples also contain vitamin C, which can reduce the severity of colds.
- There is a fair dose of potassium in an apple, which helps to keep the levels of this important chemical in your blood correctly balanced.
- Apples have something called bioflavonoids, which are really types of vitamin C. These stabilize blood vessel membranes and can help to reduce bleeding.
- Apples contain a good amount of dietary fiber which may help prevent colon cancer and even reduce the cholesterol level.
- A substance called pectin in apples also may help lower cholesterol.

So, be good to yourself today—give yourself an apple!

DOES ASPIRIN PREVENT HEART ATTACK?

Recent studies indicate that aspirin helps prevent heart attacks if taken on a daily or every-other-day basis.

Aspirin acts as a blood thinner that affects small particles in your blood called platelets. These are sticky little particles that adhere to the surface of an injured blood vessel and help you to stop bleeding if you cut yourself. When cholesterol, a waxy substance, collects on the lining of a blood vessel, the body interprets this to be an injury to that blood vessel, and it sends the platelets to stick to the surface. This results in a clot on the top of the cholesterol. If this clot becomes large enough, it shuts off the flow of blood in the vessel, and that is essentially what causes a heart attack.

Aspirin seems to impair the function of these platelets so they can't stick together and, therefore, can't form clots. The research suggests that taking one adult aspirin every other day (or perhaps daily) will keep the blood flowing freely and prevent clots.

Unfortunately, there are numerous side effects to aspirin, including stomach ulcers, excessive bleeding, and possible increased risk for hemorrhagic stroke. Also, if a regular aspirin user were to be injured in an accident or need emergency surgery, bleeding might be a more serious problem than for the non-aspirin user.

At this time, most physicians do not recommend daily aspirin for everyone. However, if you have a strong family history of heart disease or if you're in a high-risk group for heart attacks (smoking, cholesterol), you might benefit from taking aspirin as long as you have no side effects from it. A daily aspirin usually *is* recommended for people who have already had a heart attack or bypass surgery. Your doctor can help you decide if taking a daily aspirin will help you avoid heart attack.

ASPIRIN AND REYE'S SYNDROME

BEWARE OF USING ASPIRIN FOR A CHILD'S FEVER

Reye's syndrome is a serious but rare illness that can strike children recovering from chicken pox or influenza. It is associated with violent and persistent vomiting, drowsiness, and then a comatose condition with rapid breathing, stiffness, and twisting of the body. Up to 30 percent of children who get Reye's syndrome will die unless they are diagnosed early and treated. When treated, only 5 percent will have a fatal outcome. About 200 to 300 children die each year from Reye's syndrome.

Recent evidence suggests that using aspirin during a fever, especially with chicken pox or flu, may be associated with an increased incidence of Reye's syndrome. Although this is still under investigation, any child or teenager with a fever that you think needs treating should use a non-aspirin type of medication such as acetaminophen (Tylenol®). Remember that fever is not necessarily bad; it can be useful in fighting infections (see *Fever*, page 36). If the fever is under 102 degrees F and there are no significant uncomfortable side effects, it may be that no treatment is needed.

PREVENT IT WITH SIMPLE HOME EXERCISES

Improper lifting of heavy objects, poor posture, physical injury, and even poor physical fitness all contribute to back problems. Exercising is one of the best ways to prevent back problems. Try the following back-strengthening exercises:

•   The *pelvic tilt.* Lie on your back with your knees drawn up and arms at your sides. Now pull in your stomach while flattening the lower part of your back against the floor. Hold for a count of five and then relax for a count of 5.

•   The *knee hug* increases your back flexibility. Lie on your back and bring your right knee up to your chest, pulling gently on it with your hands; then lower it. Repeat with the left knee. Then raise both knees together, lowering one leg at a time.

•   *Partial sit-ups* strengthen the abdominal muscles that help support the spine. Lying on your back with both knees bent, tuck your chin in to your chest and then raise your upper body slowly with your arms at your sides, until your shoulder blades just clear the floor. Hold for a count of five and then relax back. You don't need to come all the way up to strengthen the abdominal muscles.

Don't exercise if your back is already sore! Rest it first until it feels better. Do the exercises daily, but not for at least an hour after getting up in the morning. Wait until you've been up and around for awhile and your body is warmed up and loosened up. Start with five repetitions and work up to 10. Try to keep up this exercise program. Letting your back get out of shape will make you vulnerable to problems all over again.

BEE STINGS

ALLERGIC REACTIONS CAN BE SEVERE

Spring and summer bring a multitude of stinging insects that can pose a danger during your outdoor activities.

For most people, stings from bees and wasps are only a temporary annoyance, but for some a sting can cause serious reactions and even death.

Besides the usual pain and itching from stings, people who are allergic to bee and wasp venom may experience hives, flushing, breathing problems such as wheezing or hoarseness, chest constriction, difficulty swallowing, abdominal cramps, and a sudden drop of blood pressure, shock, or even death.

How do you know if you will react severely to stings? If you reacted badly to your first sting, you will need to be careful the next time, because your reaction could become worse with each exposure. On the other hand, reacting normally to the first sting does not necessarily protect you. Some people develop sensitivity after multiple stings.

Here are some hints for avoiding bee stings.

- If you encounter a stinging insect, back away slowly. It is probably looking for pollen and won't attack you unless it is provoked.
- Keep your shoes on while walking through flower beds and low-lying plants such as clover.
- Be especially careful after a rain, when pollen is scarce and the insects are more easily excited.

If you do get stung, don't pull the stinger out. Scrape it away with your fingernail to avoid squeezing out more venom.

If you react severely to stings, it is important to seek medical attention. In the future, you may need to carry a special injection kit with you, to use immediately if a bite occurs. The kits, which are available commercially from your pharmacist with a prescription from your doctor, stop the severe reactions.

An allergist can desensitize you to bee stings. Strongly consider this option if you have even mild reactions.

BELL'S PALSY

FACIAL "DROOP" RESEMBLES STROKE

Do you know some people who look like they'd had a stroke affecting one side of the face but then recovered over the next few weeks? This facial droop or paralysis is called Bell's palsy. It involves a nerve near the front of the ear that supplies most of one side of the face. The cause of this problem, although it is thought to be a virus, is actually unknown.

The paralysis comes on rapidly, within a few hours or sometimes over a few days. The problem is usually first noticed in the morning upon waking. There is pain behind the ear and sometimes tears flow from the involved eye; the face feels numb. The most prominent feature is severe muscle weakness on the affected side of the face. The ability to taste is sometimes affected as well.

Even untreated, 80 to 85 percent of people with Bell's palsy recover completely or almost so. In a smaller number, facial weakness may persist. There may be some leftover paralysis that can affect chewing and eye blinking. Inability to blink can lead to excessive tear production.

People who are going to recover completely usually show improvement during the first two weeks, while those destined to have some permanent residual disability usually show no change for three to four months. It is difficult to predict who will and who won't improve.

Rehabilitative treatment includes electrical stimulation of the facial nerves and sometimes cortisone medication to reduce inflammation. People who have Bell's palsy should massage and exercise the face daily. Some doctors recommend chewing gum in order to have constant stimulation of the nerves. Since the

9

blink mechanism of the eye is gone, eye drops must be used to keep the eye moist. Eye protection is a must, especially outdoors, in order to keep debris out of the eye. When sleeping, the eye needs to be taped shut. This is often done with a ball of cotton and some surgical tape.

Although Bell's palsy is a frightening condition, most people recover completely. If it happens to you, make sure you see your doctor, because certain treatments and medications can promote quicker healing.

BLOOD PRESSURE

PART I—WHAT IT IS

The heart is a pump made of muscle. The first sound is the initial contraction of the heart muscle. The purpose of the contraction is to send a squirt of blood into the arteries to begin the long journey throughout the body. The second sound is the relaxation of the heart as the valves close.

As the blood is pushed through the arteries it exerts pressure—blood pressure—against the artery walls, causing them to expand and relax with the heart's rhythm. This expanding and relaxing of the arteries is what gives rise to the two numbers associated with blood pressure readings.

As the heart contracts, it pumps blood into the artery, forcing the artery to expand. The amount of force needed to expand the artery is called the "systolic" pressure. This is the top (and larger) number of a blood pressure reading.

After the blood is pumped through, the artery relaxes. The pressure that exists inside the artery while the heart rests is called the "diastolic" pressure. This is the bottom (and smaller) number of the reading.

PART II—HOW IT'S MEASURED

A sphygmomanometer is used to measure blood pressure. This includes a cuff with an air bladder inside which is pumped up to increase pressure on the arm. A pressure gauge measures how high the pressure goes.

When the doctor takes your blood pressure, he or she pumps up the cuff around your arm to above your systolic (expanding) pressure. This collapses the artery so no blood gets through. Then he or she listens with a stethoscope over the artery while slowly reducing the cuff pressure by releasing the air. The moment the pressure of the cuff drops lower than the blood's systolic pressure, the doctor will hear the sound of the first blood being pumped into the artery. The doctor immediately checks the gauge and records this as your systolic reading (top number).

As the doctor continues lowering the cuff pressure, he or she will hear the sound of blood pulsing through the artery until the cuff pressure equals the blood's diastolic (resting) pressure. Here the sound stops and a gauge reading indicates the diastolic pressure (bottom number).

If either the systolic or diastolic number is higher than normal (120/80), then arteries are too stiff. Persistently high blood pressure damages the arteries.

Occasionally, excessive nervousness can temporarily elevate blood pressure ("white coat hypertension").

Now that you know what blood pressure is and how to check it, it's important to keep track of yours, since high blood pressure is the leading cause of heart attack and stroke. If you have high blood pressure, consider getting a home blood pressure kit in order to keep better track of it. Digital kits are the most popular because they're the easiest to use. No need for a stethoscope; pressure is displayed automatically. These units are generally accurate. To check this, we have our patients bring their kits to the office to compare their reading with ours. The units provided for public use at drugstores and shopping malls tend to be less accurate, perhaps because of high use. They are best used only for screening purposes to decide whether a visit to the doctor is necessary.

HIGH BLOOD PRESSURE

NEW FINDINGS AND NORMAL LIMITS

Normal blood pressure is 120/80 (or within a range of 100-140/65-90). The American Heart Association used to suggest that blood pressure greater than 160/95 required treatment; now they regard blood pressure greater than 140/90 to be abnormal. Heart problems and stroke can develop when elevations persist above 140/90. What this means, then, is that 20 million more people than previously estimated have high blood pressure; that's one out of every four people in the United States!

If you haven't checked your blood pressure in a while, it would be a good idea to do so. If you have blood pressure problems or fluctuations, a home blood pressure kit might be best for you. These can be purchased at many drug and hospital supply stores. Taking your blood pressure often at home probably is more accurate than the isolated readings obtained in the doctor's office where some anxiety could cause the pressure to rise.

Just because you have high blood pressure doesn't mean you have to be on medication. There are several things you can do to bring your pressure down:
- Lose excess weight.
- Reduce salt intake.
- Increase physical activity and fitness.
- Reduce alcohol intake.

These simple measures might bring your pressure back to normal. Even if you need to start medication, it does not necessarily mean it is going to be a lifelong affair. If you are able to make some of the above changes in your lifestyle, you might be able to reduce or eliminate your need for the medication. Just be sure to continue taking your medication as prescribed until your doctor advises otherwise.

BOTTLED WATER

WHAT DO YOU GET FOR YOUR MONEY?

What sounds more refreshing than a cold drink of water from a bubbling mountain stream or a deep artesian well? It's the mineral content that gives such water its appealing taste. This is the "taste image" promoted by distributors of bottled water. But do you really get that taste when you buy their products?

Bottled water may or may not come from a natural spring, but it is altered before it reaches your lips.

For one thing, it is purified. One of the methods used for purification is called deionization, which removes most of the minerals from the water. In another method, called reverse osmosis, the water is forced under pressure through a plastic membrane that acts as a filter and again some minerals are removed. In some cases, some of the minerals are put back in again to give the water some taste.

Almost all the water bottled and sold in America gets ozonated. Right before it is poured into its receptacle it is injected with ozone. This is a bluish form of oxygen often used commercially as a bleaching agent and germicide. It does the same job as chlorine but it doesn't have the same aftertaste or smell. This is what gives the water a slightly bluish cast. So, although bottled water is usually pure, it may lack most minerals and have lost most of its taste.

WHAT TO EAT FOR BREAKFAST

COFFEE AND DOUGHNUTS OR NOTHING AT ALL?

Breakfast. Some love it, some leave it.

If you're standing in the kitchen trying to decide between having some junk food, in the form of coffee and doughnuts, or skipping breakfast altogether, which is better?

When it's a choice between junk food or nothing in the morning, the nod goes to nothing. Caffeine and sugar may rev up your engines, but they're going to stall out later in the morning, and you will probably be better off running on empty.

When you first wake up in the morning, your body is humming along on what is called a fasting metabolism. Since the body has been deprived of food all night, it is using stored fat for energy. Your blood sugar level may be low, but it's stable. When you throw in coffee and doughnuts, the sugar level rises significantly, perhaps giving a sense of energy. However, as the sugar comes down in the mid-morning, it leads to a feeling of loss of energy. This can interfere with your morning work performance.

The best way to coax up your morning sugar level is with some protein. This raises blood sugar in a calm, controlled way to preserve a nice, steady state of mind.

I know this might sound unusual, but I'm recommending that you try a little cottage cheese, yogurt, or even an egg (see *Yolkless Egg*, page 32) in the morning to get some protein instead of all that sugar-coated stuff that you've been wolfing down. If you simply can't eat when you get up, then skip breakfast and eat some of the above later in the morning. And, if you have time, balance off breakfast with some fruit, cereal, and even a little fat.

Consider getting up a little earlier and starting your day off right!

HOW TO FIGHT THE WINTER BLUES

Winter depression is a serious problem for many, especially after the winter holidays. Because of a combination of cold outdoor temperatures, shorter daylight hours, and little sunshine, people begin to feel tired, bored, and isolated.

Light definitely plays a part in this problem. Most of us are sensitive to long periods of grayness and dullness and lack of sunshine. Experts believe that a lack of sunlight affects a portion of the brain called the pineal gland. This causes biological changes in some people, resulting in moodiness and depression. Darkness and cold weather, which keep most of us indoors where social interaction and activity are limited, can lead to feelings of restlessness and boredom and sometimes to even more serious problems, such as excessive alcohol use and overeating.

The best medicine for winter depression is to take part in some outdoor activity, even if it's just walking for short periods of time. Some exposure to sunlight is essential.

Winter does not have to be a downer. Keeping yourself busy and getting plenty of exercise, along with your daily dose of sunshine, will help you feel better about yourself and the world around you!

CARPAL TUNNEL SYNDROME

DO YOUR HANDS "GO TO SLEEP" AT NIGHT?

Have you ever awakened at night with your thumb and first two fingers tingling and throbbing? Have you ever had trouble writing or opening jars? If so, you may have carpal tunnel syndrome.

With this disorder, the median nerve, which comes down the forearm and through the wrist to the thumb and first two fingers and half of the third finger, becomes trapped between the ligaments and tendons in the wrist because of swelling or scar tissue. The swelling can press on the nerve and cause the numbness and tingling. The pain is not limited to the hand; it can travel up into the forearm and shoulder. If the symptoms are ignored too long, there can be permanent loss of feeling in those fingers, as well as loss of muscle strength.

This disease can affect one hand or both, but it usually starts in the dominant hand, the one you use the most. The symptoms often occur at night or while reading a book or newspaper. They can be relieved by shaking the hand vigorously. Sleeping intensifies the problem because the tissues in the wrist normally swell somewhat at night. Most cases are caused by overuse of the wrist or excessive stress to the wrist tissues. People who use their hands in their work are subject to this. It has occurred in computer operators who rest their wrists against the edge of the desk leading to damaged tissue; wrist guards for the edge of computer desks have sometimes been helpful. In addition, this syndrome tends to occur frequently during pregnancy or in persons with some types of arthritis. Women seem to be affected more often than men.

The diagnosis can usually be made with a simple test done in the doctor's office. Occasionally, an electrical stimulation test may be necessary. Bending your wrist at 90 degrees to the forearm and holding it in that position for several seconds can sometimes produce the symptoms; if that happens, then the likelihood of your having carpal tunnel syndrome is high.

Treatment can be as simple as avoiding activities that aggravate the condition. In addition, a splint can be applied to the wrist to hold it up and take the pressure off the nerve, especially at night. If the splint doesn't work, cortisone drugs can be injected into the area to reduce swelling. Surgery might be necessary to release the pressure around the nerve. If you think you have this problem, consult your physician. If treated early, carpal tunnel syndrome can be completely cured.

HEART ATTACK PAIN IS NOT ALWAYS "PAINFUL"

Identifying the source of chest pain and trying to determine if it's caused by cardiac disease is often very difficult. That's because chest pain from the heart is often not "painful." It's better described as a pressure, tightness, or heaviness. Sometimes, it's even associated with gas or nausea and can easily be mistaken for indigestion. It's probably more accurate to refer to it as a chest "discomfort" rather than a chest "pain."

This chest discomfort travels not only down the left arm (which is the most commonly described) but also down both arms, into the back, and quite characteristically into the neck and jaw. Most people are not aware of these unusual locations for the pain and often ignore the symptoms. Some even think they have a dental problem when the pain radiates to the jaw. Sweating in the upper half of the body is also a fairly characteristic sign associated with cardiac pain.

Typically, cardiac pain is not relieved with change of position; deep breathing, twisting, or turning do *not* seem to make it any better or worse. *Muscular* types of pain, which are less serious, *are* affected by those particular motions.

It is often difficult even for a physician to be certain of what is causing the chest pain, and whether it truly represents cardiac problems. If you are in doubt, seek medical help, or go to the nearest emergency room. Remember, it's better to make an unnecessary trip to the hospital than to miss the beginning of a heart attack.

CHEWING TOBACCO AND SNUFF

STILL A TEENAGE PROBLEM

Young people are still chewing tobacco and using snuff. Many are influenced by seeing their favorite athletes using it. While most of us are aware of the dangers of smoking cigarettes, we are not as aware that the same dangers exist with chewing tobacco and snuff.

Chewing tobacco is a mixture of tobacco and molasses and is chewed by stuffing a golfball-sized wad between the cheek and the teeth. It is "dipped" by placing a "pinch" of it between the lower lip and gum. In both cases, the nicotine and tobacco is absorbed through the gums and into the blood stream just like any other drug. It is habit-forming, and users can develop white patches in the mouth called leukoplakia. About 5 percent of cases of leukoplakia develop into cancer of the mouth. Cancer of this area of the head and neck can be devastating and disfiguring.

Chewing tobacco and snuff are not safe replacements for smoking. It is simply trading one danger for another!

CHICKEN SOUP

IT HAS SOME MEDICINAL MERIT

Did your grandmother ever recommend chicken soup when you had a cold? It's an old-fashioned remedy that does have some merit to it. Researchers at the University of Florida tested whether there was any medical benefit to chicken soup. They found that eating chicken soup causes an increase in nasal secretions that wash out the viruses. It is important to remove these secretions by blowing the nose, since the shorter the time the virus is in the nose, the quicker the cold goes away.

When chicken soup was compared with hot water, the researchers found the amount of mucus production from the nose was much greater with chicken soup than with the hot water. So there is apparently something in the chicken soup itself that seems to help remove the viruses from the nose by stimulating free flow of secretions.

Many cold sufferers reach for drugstore remedies, not chicken soup. It's important to limit use of severe drying agents such as cold tablets when you have a cold. They might make you feel better, but they also reduce the flow of secretions and can prolong the cold by allowing the virus to live and multiply in those secretions. If you have to go to work and the cold is interfering with your performance, antihistamines may help—as long as they don't make you drowsy. But, if you are able to stay home, it might be better just to let your nose run and help it along with a little chicken soup!

CIGAR AND PIPE SMOKING

AN ALTERNATIVE TO CIGARETTES?

Are cigars and pipes less of a health risk than cigarettes?

The levels of nicotine and carbon monoxide in the blood in cigar and pipe smokers may be lower than in cigarette smokers, but they are still significantly above normal. Even though pipe and cigar smokers may not inhale, some of the nicotine and other noxious substances are still absorbed directly from the mucous membranes and lining of the mouth. And if you switch from cigarettes to either a pipe or cigars, your tendency to inhale will be much greater than if you simply started out with a pipe or cigars. In fact, "converted" cigarette smokers who unconsciously inhale the pipe or cigar smoke have even *higher* levels of nicotine and carbon monoxide than cigarette smokers. Also, the risk of mouth and lip cancer is much higher from cigars and pipes than from cigarettes.

The ideal is to stop using all forms of tobacco.

CLAUDICATION

LEG CRAMPS WHILE WALKING

Walking is an ideal exercise, but for some people it can cause pain in the hips and legs. Although the pain is often confused with arthritis, it might represent a more serious problem. This particular pain is caused by partial blockage of the arteries to the leg, usually due to a build-up of fat or cholesterol. It is referred to as "intermittent claudication." This build-up reduces the blood flow and causes the legs to ache or cramp during exercise. The most common sites for claudication are the hips, thighs, calves, and arch of the foot. Other symptoms include overall fatigue and weakness of the legs. Typically, people who have this problem are able to walk a specific distance, such as one to two blocks, after which the cramps and aching set in. Then, after a brief rest, they can resume walking. Although some mistakenly interpret this to be arthritis, it is actually a circulation problem.

Claudication can easily be diagnosed and treated by your physician. Some of the following measures may be recommended: First, stop smoking, since smokers face twice the risk of developing this problem. Second, take care of your feet, and wear shoes that protect them, since injuries to the foot will heal very poorly because of the abnormal circulation. And third, believe it or not, walk. Walking is good for your circulation, providing you stop and rest as soon as it becomes painful.

Medication or surgery might be necessary to improve the blood flow. If you think you have this condition, it's important to see your physician, both to confirm the diagnosis and to obtain adequate treatment.

WHEN TO TREAT—WHEN TO SEE THE DOCTOR

Weather doesn't cause colds. But the number of colds does seem to increase with sharp changes in temperature—either up or down. You're more susceptible to colds when you're tired, under emotional stress, or recovering from an illness.

You can cut down on your chances of catching a cold by reducing stress, eating well, sleeping enough, and washing your hands often.

Experiments at an army base showed that colds were reduced considerably when infected people wiped their hands and noses with iodine-soaked tissues before entering public rooms. Hands are probably the major way that colds are passed to others! I'm not recommending iodine-soaked tissues—just wash your hands frequently to avoid "handing off" your cold to others.

There is no cure for the common cold. Nearly 100 cold-causing viruses have been identified so far, and some of these viruses can change forms quickly, rendering the body's antibody system useless against the new strain.

Most colds run their course in one to two weeks. You can relieve your symptoms with some simple home remedies like chicken soup (see page 18), plenty of fluids, vitamin C, and nonprescription drugs.

But remember that all medications, whether prescription or not, merit respect. It's important to know what you're taking and whether it can have an effect on any other disease or problem that you have, such as hypertension.

Sometimes colds are a symptom of more serious illness. If you have a cold you need to call your doctor if:

- You seem unusually ill.
- You want to take a nonprescription product and are already taking a prescribed medication.
- You have a chronic disease.

- You have trouble breathing.
- You have a sore throat with swollen glands and no other typical cold symptoms.
- You have a lingering headache.
- You have symptoms that don't fade after a week.
- You have a sputum-producing cough.
- . You have an earache.

It may be difficult to remember all of these guidelines, so—if in doubt, contact your physician.

OVER-THE-COUNTER COLD MEDICATIONS

WHICH ONE TO CHOOSE?

Many of us head for a drugstore at the first sign of a cold. But even over-the-counter medication has to be taken with care. Mixing medications or taking too much of one can make you feel worse than you already do. The five categories of over-the-counter cold medications are analgesics, antihistamines, decongestants, expectorants, and antitussives. Each of these is useful for a specific symptom.

Analgesics: These are basically pain killers, often of the aspirin or acetaminophen type, taken specifically for the aches and pains common at the onset of a cold. They will not cure your cold. And if you take them throughout the entire course of your cold, you could mask a fever that might be an indication of a more serious underlying bacterial infection. If you can tolerate the aches and pains, don't use analgesics. And keep track of any fever that persists. It should be reported to your doctor.

Antihistamines: These are used for drying the secretions of a cold and for preventing sneezing and watery, itchy eyes. Beware—they can also cause drowsiness. They may be sold in combination with a decongestant.

Decongestants: These drugs help dry up the secretions in the nose or lungs. They come in tablets or capsules or sometimes in a nasal spray or drops. These medications are not recommended for people with high blood pressure, and they can cause jitteriness and irritability in others. These are often sold in combination with an antihistamine, but they can be purchased separately and are useful when you want to avoid drowsiness.

Expectorants: These agents help to loosen phlegm so it can be coughed up. Increasing humidity and drinking lots of fluids will probably do the same thing.

Antitussives: These are used to suppress coughs, especially dry, scratchy coughs. They may allow you to function better at work and to get some sleep at night, but usually it is better to cough the material out, if possible. Sometimes just increasing the humidity, especially at night, will also help the cough.

Before taking any medication, read the label. Make it your business to know which medications you're taking, what they're supposed to do, and what the possible side effects are.

COLITIS

INFLAMMATORY BOWEL DISEASE

Inflammatory bowel disease (IBD) is a general term for a group of chronic inflammatory disorders of uncertain cause involving the gastrointestinal tract. It strikes most often between the ages of 15 and 35 and is more common among Caucasian and Jewish people than others. Family tendency is a factor in some cases.

There are two forms of IBD: ulcerative colitis and Crohn's disease.

Abdominal pain and bloody diarrhea, sometimes with fever and weight loss, are the major symptoms of ulcerative colitis. The symptoms are caused by inflammation and bleeding of the lining of the colon. If the condition continues for a long time, the colon can become scarred and deformed.

Most persons with ulcerative colitis have mild to moderate diseases of an intermittent nature that can be managed without hospitalization. More rarely, the disease can involve the entire colon and cause severe bloody diarrhea. In such cases, there is risk that the colon might become dilated or even perforated. This is a medical emergency.

Crohn's disease typically strikes a young man or woman and causes fatigue, variable weight loss, and abdominal pain. There may also be fever and diarrhea, often without blood. Intestinal obstruction is possible, as well as fistula formation (an abnormal connection between two segments of the bowel). Sometimes the examining physicians mistake Crohn's disease for acute appendicitis.

Both forms of IBD commonly include a nondeforming type of arthritis especially involving the knees, ankles, and wrists. There are reports of increased incidence of malignancy developing in Crohn's disease and even more often in ulcerative colitis.

Anti-inflammatory agents, sulfa-type products, and cortisone preparations are used to treat IBD. Up to one-fourth of persons with ulcerative colitis require surgery, while nearly three-fourths of Crohn's disease sufferers will need at least one operation in the course of their illness.

IBD can be serious. But with prompt diagnosis and treatment, a normal lifestyle is possible.

If any of these symptoms fit abnormalities you have, consult your physician.

COLON CANCER

A SIMPLE HOME TEST FOR THIS MAJOR KILLER

Next to skin cancer in men and breast cancer in women, cancer of the colon and rectum are the most common tumors and can affect up to 1 in 4 persons over age 40.

Evidence suggests that diets high in cholesterol, especially from beef fat and eggs, (see *Yolkless Egg,* page32) play a role in stimulating production of cancer of the colon, especially in families prone to this type of tumor.

Foods with high fiber content act in just the opposite way and can reduce the incidence of colon cancer. This could be due to the ability of a high-fiber diet to speed the passage of all substances through the intestine, minimizing their contact with the intestinal wall.

To avoid colorectal cancer, use eggs sparingly, trim the fat off your meat, and take enough fiber or bran with your breakfast cereal every day (2 to 3 heaping tablespoonsful) to keep your bowels moving easily.

Prevention is of prime importance in avoiding this killer cancer. Over three-quarters of the victims of this type of tumor can be cured and will be able to return to their normal lives if it is detected early enough. One of the most effective screening methods for this type of cancer is a stool test that checks for hidden blood. You can get a home testing kit for blood in the stool from your physician or hospital clinic or even from the drugstore. The test is simple and can be done at home in a few moments without help. Stool samples should be obtained on three separate days once a year. If any sample is positive for blood, the person is advised to avoid red meat, iron-containing medicines and vitamin C for three days and repeat the test (since all of these can cause a false-positive test). Should any of these second-round samples be positive for blood, the person is advised to visit a physician for investigation of the problem. Bowel x-rays will probably be necessary.

The minor inconvenience of checking three stool specimens a year is insignificant compared with the possibility of missing an early tumor. If you have any questions on how to do this, be sure to contact your physician.

COUGH MEDICATIONS

WHICH ONE SHOULD YOU CHOOSE?

What can you do about a nagging cough that interferes with your daily routine or your sleep? Cough medications are of questionable benefit. Even expectorants, which are supposed to loosen the mucus, don't always help.

Cough suppressants work on the part of the brain that controls the cough reflex. Some experts feel that when we cough we are doing so for a reason—to raise phlegm—and it might not be a good idea to suppress that response.

Both antihistamines and decongestants may thicken the mucus and make it dryer and more difficult to cough up.

Cough drops are made mostly of sugar. They have some soothing action and may contain some of the above-mentioned ingredients, but they really offer nothing else.

What about home remedies? Some holistic remedies include putting a drop of honey on the back of the tongue (which is supposed to help loosen the mucus), increasing fluid intake (by drinking fruit juices and other liquids), eating chicken soup, and using humidifiers. All of these measures can help relieve your cough.

Coughing, especially if you are coughing something up, is a healthy way to clear your bronchial tubes. Use a cough suppressant during the day only if the cough interferes with your work, or at night if you can't get to sleep. Remember, the suppressants contain mild narcotics and can cause drowsiness.

Usually it's better to stick with the natural remedies, as described above, and to cough up the mucus and phlegm, since this material contains some of the germs. But if your cough persists for more than a week or if you are having trouble breathing, it's time to visit the doctor.

CPR AND THE HEIMLICH MANEUVER

EVERYONE SHOULD KNOW HOW!

Cardiopulmonary resuscitation (CPR) is an essential lifesaving technique that we all should know how to do. Persons whose heart and lungs have stopped need to have circulation restarted within four to six minutes to prevent brain damage. The following are some guidelines for both CPR and for the Heimlich maneuver (which is used when people are choking).

The first step is to determine if the victim is unconscious. If there is no response from the victim, always call for help. Then clear the victim's airway (open the mouth) and check for breathing by listening closely to his or her mouth and watching the chest for movement. If the person is not breathing, give four quick, full breaths, using mouth-to-mouth resuscitation. (Each breath lasts one to two seconds). This procedure requires some training, but in a true emergency, some breath—even given by an inexperienced person—is better than no breath at all!

Next, check for a pulse (feel the neck with two fingers just along either side of the windpipe). If there is a pulse and no breathing, give only mouth-to-mouth resuscitation, about every five seconds. If there is no pulse and no breathing, get emergency medical help, and then begin a series of chest compressions, using the heel of your hand, over the breastbone (sternum), again followed by quick full breaths with mouth-to-mouth resuscitation. Continue checking for the pulse and breathing and wait for help.

Another well-known lifesaving technique is called the Heimlich maneuver. It is used on choking victims. The universal sign of choking is to put both hands around your throat. This signals others that you cannot speak and are choking. If the victim is not able to breathe or speak, you need to call for help and you have about four minutes to clear the victim's air passageway. Do this by standing behind the victim and wrapping your arms around him or her, with your fist positioned in the upper abdomen. Using your fist, pull toward yourself with quick upward thrusts into the victim's abdomen. Keep repeating this until the object is expelled out of the mouth. Essentially, you're pushing into the abdomen to expel air through the lungs, in the hope of pushing the foreign object out of the breathing tube.

It is worthwhile to get training in these measures. They can be harmful if not done properly. Certainly, if anyone in your family has heart or lung trouble, someone in the household should know these techniques.

LOSE WEIGHT—IMPROVE TYPE II DIABETES

BODY WEIGHT IS ONE OF THE MAJOR FACTORS IN CONTROLLING BLOOD SUGAR LEVELS

There are two forms of diabetes. Type I is referred to as juvenile or insulin-dependent diabetes. It strikes at a young age and is associated with a lack of insulin production in the pancreas. The more common form of diabetes occurs in adults and is called Type II, or noninsulin-dependent diabetes. This is usually a genetic disorder in which the body handles both carbohydrates and fats in an abnormal way. In addition, some tissues, such as muscle, become insensitive to the effects of insulin. As a means of compensation, more insulin is produced in order to maintain a normal level of blood sugar. Early on in the disease, this leads to an accumulation of body fat which aggravates the problem because fat increases the body's resistance to insulin. So, a vicious cycle is set up. Ultimately, as the compensation system fails, the blood glucose levels begin to rise and diabetes becomes severe enough to cause symptoms.

High levels of glucose affect the lining of blood vessels, causing them to be distorted and even fragile. Ultimately severe vascular problems such as stroke, heart attack, kidney failure, and deterioration of the retina of the eye can occur. However, there are things a person with diabetes can do to improve this condition. And probably the most important is to control body weight.

Physical activity is useful in combatting diabetes for two reasons. Exercise increases the muscles' sensitivity to insulin, allowing a normal blood sugar to be maintained with less secretion of insulin. And exercise helps keep body fat from accumulating. Less body fat means greater sensitivity to insulin and therefore more normal levels of blood sugar.

A proper diabetic diet can help you reach and maintain your ideal body weight. The diet includes a good balance of protein, fat, and carbohydrates along with a reduction in calories. In addition, the diet should include significant portions of complex carbohydrates. These carbohydrates are digested more slowly and therefore don't cause a rapid rise in the blood sugar. Included in this group of foods are pastas, fruits, and vegetables. With these dietary changes, some adults with Type II diabetes can control their blood sugar without medication.

Even if you can't completely control your blood sugar with exercise and weight loss, having to take pills is no cause for despair. And good control of blood sugar helps prevent the vascular complications of this disease mentioned earlier. Sometimes taking the pills for a short period will buy time until a weight loss and exercise program can begin to work. It's possible that with adequate exercise and diet a person with Type II diabetes will be able to stop taking diabetes pills or insulin shots. However, don't do this on your own. Make sure your doctor checks your progress regularly and agrees with any decision to change treatment.

YOUR MEDICAL APPOINTMENT

HOW TO GET MORE OUT OF IT

A doctor's appointment represents not only a personal and medical encounter, but also a business relationship. It's important that you get the most out of it. Here are some hints to improve your next visit:

- When you set your appointment, indicate the type of problem you have and how much extra time you may need to discuss it.
- Bring a written list of your symptoms and questions you want to ask.
- Especially if this is a first visit, bring a list of what medications you are on, your family medical history, and any important events in your own medical history such as previous hospitalizations, surgeries, or allergies.
- If possible, do some advance reading and research about your condition in order to help you ask better questions.
- . Take along a note pad so you can jot down important information.
- . If you don't understand what was said, ask the physician to repeat the explanation until it is clear to you.
- If you have not responded to a previous treatment, ask your doctor if he or she will consider an alternative. And don't be embarrassed to discuss side effects of medications, including those that might affect sexual function.

Remember, doctors see many patients every day. Those who show interest and have good questions about their conditions will often receive more attention and better answers!

IT CAN BE ASSOCIATED WITH ARTHRITIS

Dry eyes are a very aggravating problem for as many as 7 million Americans. If you are a woman over 60, you're a prime candidate for this particular problem. The difficulty occurs because the tear glands dry up, sometimes permanently, reducing the amount of lubrication to the eye. The white of the eye then gets irritated, red, and swollen. You may have a "sand-in-the-eye" feeling. This disease can also be accompanied by dry mouth, irritated joints, and even a drying up of some of the digestive juices.

One cause of this problem is rheumatoid arthritis, often associated with a drying up of the salivary and tear glands (Sjogren's syndrome). Quite often, however, no cause is found.

If you think you have this problem, it's important to see your doctor so he or she can prescribe a lubricant (artificial tears) to use several times a day. Vitamin supplements including A, B, C, and E have also been helpful for some people. In addition, the following guidelines are recommended:

- •. Use only white tissues since dyes in colored tissues might irritate the eye.
- • Use a humidifier at home.
- • Wear sunglasses to shield and protect your eyes.
- • Avoid fumes from strong chemical cleaners such as oven cleaners.

EAR WAX

WHAT CAN YOU DO ABOUT IT?

You have probably heard the old saying, "Never put anything smaller than your elbow into your ear." It's old, but it's true. So what should you do if your ear is plugged up and wax is the culprit?

There is a purpose to ear wax. It traps dust and other particles and protects the eardrum. When it builds up enough to block the ear canal and impair your hearing, here is what to do. You could see your doctor and obtain an ear wax softener by prescription, or you can do the following: Using an eyedropper, drop a small amount of baby oil, mineral oil, or glycerine into the ear twice a day for several days. Next, using a bulb syringe, flush the ear canal with body-temperature water. Turn your head to the side to drain it all out. Then, insert an eyedropperful of rubbing alcohol into the ear and drain this out. The alcohol absorbs water and helps to dry the ear canal.

Do not try this if your ear is painful, tender, or draining. If you have any doubts about the condition of your ear, see your doctor or an ear, nose, and throat specialist.

EGGS AND CHOLESTEROL

TRY THE "YOLKLESS EGG"

I'm sure all of you are aware of the problems with cholesterol and how you need to reduce the consumption of this substance in your diet. Perhaps you've also read my earlier health tip suggesting that it's better to have a high-protein breakfast in order to avoid the mid-morning slump (see *Breakfast* page 14). Many people like to eat eggs for breakfast, and they become discouraged when told they shouldn't have more than two to four eggs per week, including eggs used in cooking and baking. Well, how can you get protein in the morning without eggs?

Here's a simple solution. Remember this about eggs: There's lots of protein both in the white and in the yolk—but all of the cholesterol is in the yolk. I don't mean to minimize the importance of the egg yolk, because it does contain most of the essential amino acids that are important building blocks in the body. However, if you'd like to have more eggs and avoid the cholesterol, here's all you have to do. After you crack open the egg, simply remove the yolk, poach the remaining white portion, and you will have a high protein breakfast with absolutely no cholesterol. Add a little pepper or Parmesan cheese for taste. If you include a piece of whole-wheat toast and orange juice, you'll have a perfect breakfast.

The next time you go out for breakfast, order a yolkless egg. Not only will your friends be impressed, but you won't be adding to your cholesterol.

EXERCISE

DO YOU NEED TO WARM UP AND STRETCH?

The value of warming up or stretching before exercise still remains controversial. Aggressive stretching exercises done before you are properly warmed up can injure muscles that are tight and cold and therefore don't stretch easily. Some experts believe stretching is more properly done *after* exercising.

It's more important to warm up than to stretch before exercising. You don't absolutely need to stretch, but you do need to warm up a little before you start. Of course, you need to warm up very well if you are going to do any aggressive exercising, such as racing or competitive swimming. The easiest way to warm up is to use the muscles that you are about to use in your activity in a light and easy fashion, and then gradually increase the pace. In other words, walk before jogging, jog before running, throw easy before throwing hard.

My conclusion: Stretching is optional, but the warm-up is essential, especially if you're over 40.

EXERTION IN COLD WEATHER

SOME PRECAUTIONS ARE NECESSARY FOR EVERYBODY

In some parts of the country, winter can bring bitterly cold weather. Is it safe to exercise, walk, shovel snow, or even be out in very cold temperatures?

Cold air alone, even when you are at rest, can alter your heart rate. It can also increase your blood pressure and reduce the amount of oxygen going to your heart. Persons with lung or cardiac conditions should not needlessly venture out when the wind-chill factor is below 25 degrees. Even perfectly healthy people need to take great caution when the wind chill factor drops to minus 20.

It isn't just cold temperatures that stress your body in winter. There's an extra measure of challenge in any outdoor winter activity. Walking through snow requires considerably more energy than walking on firm surfaces. Shoveling heavy snow for 10 minutes is equivalent to running for 10 minutes at 10 miles per hour! In addition, wearing bulky winter clothing restricts movement and makes whatever you're doing more difficult.

If you must go out in very cold weather, dress in layered clothing, and keep it as comfortably fitting as possible. If you have cardiac or lung problems, cover your nose and mouth in extremely cold temperatures. Cold air hitting this area of the face causes constriction of the blood vessels and can result in a rise in blood pressure. This makes the heart work harder. You will be expending extra energy, so you will need to pace yourself accordingly.

ARE YOU DESTINED TO BE OBESE?

It seems like everyone is trying to lose weight, and we each have a favorite diet to accomplish this. Unfortunately, not many of them work well. In the long run, diet failures outnumber successes by a very large margin. Only 10 percent of dieters are able to maintain their weight loss for any extended period of time. That's a 90 percent failure rate!

Some people feel there is a genetically controlled system in the brain that dictates how much fat your body should carry—a sort of "set point" or thermostat which, when you try to go under it by dieting, simply causes you to feel hungry all the time. You end up eating more until you go back to your former weight. This stable weight is often easily maintained without any conscious effort on your part. Your stable weight is the one that you usually return to after either dieting or overeating.

A study that tracked the weight of 4,000 sets of male twins has added strong evidence to the genetic or set point theory. This study, conducted on identical and non-identical twins, showed that from age 20 to 45 the identical twins were twice as likely to have the same level of obesity compared with non-identical twins.

As we get older, we seem to gain weight easier, perhaps because of some change in the metabolism or maybe a change in the set point. Of course, reduction of exercise and activity might also have something to do with it. The only thing that seems to alter this set point effectively is adding *exercise* to your dieting. So, if you want to lose weight and be able to keep it off, you must do some sort of exercise, even if it is only a brisk walk.

Whether this set point theory will end up to be true or not, I'm not sure. But it certainly is a good idea for anyone who needs to be concerned about excess weight to eat a little less and exercise a little more.

FEVER

FRIEND OR FOE?

There has always been some confusion about the true significance of a fever and whether it should be treated. Recent medical evidence suggests that a fever is more friend than foe. In fact, many experts believe a fever by itself is not necessarily harmful.

The body temperature is regulated by the brain, and when bacteria or viruses enter the bloodstream the brain sends a signal for the body to get hotter. Recent research shows that not only are many drugs more effective at higher body temperatures, but white blood cells and antibodies can fight infection more efficiently. However, if the body gets too hot (above 104.5 degrees F), the fever needs to be brought down, since dehydration and convulsions could result, especially in children.

Really, then, the only reason to reduce a mild fever (less than 102 degrees F) is to relieve the discomfort and associated aches.

When should you call a doctor about a fever?
- If it's in a child less than six months old.
- If it's in a person 65 years of age or older.
- If there is a serious illness at the same time.
- If there are any cardiac problems.
- If the temperature is over 102 degrees F.

In summary, if you or your child's temperature is under 102 degrees F and there are no other problems, it may not be necessary to treat the fever. If you do decide to treat, you should use acetaminophen instead of aspirin, especially in children or teenagers, since there is a possibility of aspirin causing a serious and often fatal liver problem called Reye's syndrome (see page 6).

IS IT WORTH MODIFYING YOUR DIET?

High-fiber diets are touted as a possible means of improving our health by lowering cholesterol, preventing colon cancer, and even improving diabetes. The question is, does this really work, and how does one go about increasing fiber in the diet?

Natural sources of dietary fiber are best. These include whole- grain products, fruits, vegetables, and legumes. The fiber content of these plant foods is not affected or broken down by our digestive enzymes and therefore passes virtually unchanged through the intestines and into the colon.

There is recent evidence that a high-fiber diet may discourage colon cancer. It could be that fiber helps to clear the colon of substances that are changed by the normal bacteria in the colon into cancer-promoting chemicals. This may occur by increasing the size of the stool and speeding the elimination of these chemicals into the stool. It could be, however, that these high-fiber diets discourage colon cancer simply because they are generally low in fat. (Diets rich in animal fat do promote colon cancer.)

Fiber improves colon function by increasing the weight and size of the stool. Therefore, it may reduce the chance of developing diverticular disease (small pockets that develop in the colon, probably resulting from poor bowel habits).

Some literature suggests that dietary fiber, especially in the form of oat bran, may help to lower blood cholesterol by preventing reabsorption of bile acids from the small intestine. Bile acids are responsible for cholesterol absorption. In addition, pectin, beans, and peas also have this desirable effect. Even commercially available psyllium seeds, which are used to prevent constipation (Metamucil, Effersyllium), may also have this effect.

Some experts speculate that high-fiber diets also reduce absorption of sugar. Therefore it's feasible that fiber may reduce the need for insulin or other anti-diabetic drugs.

It's generally recommended to have an intake of about 37 grams, or one and one-third ounces, of dietary fiber each day. This can most easily be obtained from natural sources such as whole grain breads, potatoes, fruits, vegetables, whole-grain cereals, bran muffins, and snack foods like nuts and popcorn.

Dietary supplements (high-fiber cereals, fiber pills, etc.) are not necessarily needed unless your normal diet does not contain adequate amounts of the above-mentioned food types.

If you do increase the fiber in your diet, do it gradually. Your body needs time to adjust and, at first, it might cause some increased gas formation and mild abdominal discomfort.

A balanced, moderate increase in the natural fiber in your diet is the best approach, and it may even increase the odds of avoiding some medical problems.

GENERIC DRUGS

ARE THEY A SAFE ALTERNATIVE?

It can take many years and millions of dollars to prepare a new drug for sale to the general public. Therefore, the firm that develops a new drug wants to protect its investment. While the patent for a drug is in effect, no one else can distribute it. Once the patent expires, other companies can market the drug using their own brand names. These drugs are called multiple source or generic drugs.

The question is, does the company that produced the drug first produce it any better than those who begin after the patent expires? Most generic drugs are just as effective as the originals, but there are exceptions. It's important to remember that the active ingredients of a generic drug must be the same as the original. If that's true, then why is it that some generic drugs have a different effect on the body? The answer is the presence of "inactive" ingredients. They can vary widely and the effect they can have is just not clear.

Here is my advice: Rather than shopping for price alone, find a pharmacy you can trust. They can help with the decision. Don't be afraid to ask your doctor for a recommendation, and if you have been taking a particular brand drug for a long-standing condition, don't change without first checking with your physician.

The issue of generic drugs is not new. However, it has become more important lately because more generic drugs than ever are on the market. The most important advice I can give on this issue is not to make the decision based solely on cost.

GLAUCOMA

PREVENTION IS ESSENTIAL; A CURE IS POSSIBLE

Glaucoma is a very common disease of the eye that occurs in thousands of people usually over the age of 40. Unfortunately, it may not have any symptoms and can go unrecognized for years before it progresses to rapid loss of vision.

The eye chamber is bathed in a watery fluid that flows through the eye. If the outflow of this fluid is blocked, then the fluid cannot escape and pressure builds up. This pressure cuts off the blood supply to the optic nerve located in the back of the eye, leading ultimately to blindness.

It's very important that you have the pressure in your eyes measured routinely. This can be done on a yearly basis using a device called a tonometer. This simple procedure can be done by your physician, an ophthalmologist, or an optometrist. While you are lying down, a drop of anesthetic is put into each eye and the tonometer is then placed on the cornea; this registers the pressure inside the eye. Currently, more sophisticated devices are used to measure this pressure; a puff of air from a special device can also measure the pressure in your eyes without the need for any local anesthesia.

Remember, if you are over 40 it's very important to have this done on an annual basis. This condition is correctable. Your vision is too precious to ignore this periodic check-up.

GOUTY ARTHRITIS

WATCHING YOUR DIET CAN HELP

Gout is sometimes perceived as a consequence of the excesses—of "the good life." Actually, gout is a form of arthritis. It's caused by accumulation of uric acid in the blood—either from overproduction or from poor excretion through the kidneys. Crystals of this uric acid accumulate in the joints, causing inflammation and arthritic pain. These crystals can cause knobby-looking lumps in the skin. They can also form kidney stones.

If you already have a tendency toward gout, then eating a diet that's too high in proteins or over-indulging in alcohol can aggravate the problem. Even certain types of stress (heart attack, severe illnesses) can precipitate a severe, red, swollen joint, which typically occurs in the big toe area. Fortunately, this pain responds quite well to medication, especially if treatment is started in the first day or so of an attack.

Gout can be diagnosed either by taking a blood test or a small sample of fluid from the inflamed joint. Some people have to take medicine on a daily basis in order to keep their uric acid level low enough to prevent these arthritis attacks.

HALITOSIS

DON'T WAIT FOR YOUR FRIENDS TO TELL YOU

Nobody likes to talk about bad breath, but it's an important medical and personal problem. What are the causes of bad breath? Unhealthy gums are a common cause. Various bacteria build up on the gums and, essentially, you're blowing air over something that doesn't smell very good. That's why it's important to gently brush your gums. Of course, clean teeth make a difference too. But one of the most important sources of halitosis is a filmy tongue. It's important to gently brush your tongue in the morning, as well as your teeth and gums. If you brush all three of these areas, you will eliminate most unpleasant breath odor.

But what about when this doesn't work? Another cause of halitosis is abnormal digestion. You may have to be careful about certain foods. Tobacco and alcohol don't help the breath situation either. Some mouthwashes contain alcohol, which may kill germs for about a two-hour period, but sometimes allows them to grow back faster than before!

So what's a foul mouth to do? Some suggestions:
- Brush your teeth at least twice a day.
- Gently brush the tongue at the same time as the teeth.
- Avoid excess sugar, white flour, and caffeine.
- Go easy on the alcohol.
- Regard smoking as a one-way ticket to loneliness.

HANGOVER

TREATMENT CAN BE DANGEROUS

No one is really sure what the most effective treatment for a hangover is. Many people use the nonprescription pain killer acetaminophen to relieve some of the symptoms. Acetaminophen is most popularly known as Tylenol® but is available under other brand names. It's used like aspirin, but unlike aspirin it can pose problems for heavy drinkers.

Alcohol causes acetaminophen to break down in the body in a way that produces chemicals that are poisonous to the liver. These poisons can cause liver inflammation that can result in death due to liver failure. Those who regularly drink large amounts of alcohol are at greater than normal risk. Experts recommend that people who consume three or four drinks in one day (beer, wine, or alcohol) should never take more than 2 grams of acetaminophen (8 regular-strength pills or caplets) per day. It would be a good idea to reduce the drinking as well!

HAY FEVER

SOME NEW TIPS ON PREVENTION

With the season of budding flowers and new-mown grass, comes the unpleasant and often dreaded allergic nasal syndrome called hay fever. Who hasn't seen or experienced that stuffy nose and those red, itching, watery eyes? Often it's difficult to know what the cause of the allergy really is.

Summertime attacks that begin about 5:30 to 8:30 (both morning and evening) are probably due to tree or grass pollen. They don't happen earlier in the day because the morning dew damps the pollen dust and keeps it out of the air. This contrasts with attacks that occur indoors year round, which are more likely due to house dust or pet dander. Mold sensitivity, on the other hand, is worse during damp, rainy weather; it can also be triggered by air blown into your face from a car's air conditioning unit or a room humidifier. One of the most common allergies is triggered by grass pollen, which is usually brought on by mowing the lawn. Grass allergy is thought to be caused not only by the blades of grass and the weeds themselves but also by the molds that are deposited on them.

The best treatment is to avoid exposure to the triggering substance and to reduce its concentration in your surroundings as much as possible. There isn't much one can do about pollen except stay indoors, especially from 5:30 to 8:30 a.m. and p.m. Breathe through your nose (it acts as a filter) and use a pollen mask when working in the yard. Wash your hair at bedtime to remove the accumulated pollen of the day.

In the case of mold, avoidance involves drying up damp basements, changing filters in air conditioners, cleaning humidifiers regularly, spraying with Lysol®, and keeping closets dry with a constantly lit bulb. Getting the mold out of the car's air conditioner can be difficult and usually requires a mechanic's help.

When measures such as these fail to provide relief, help can be obtained using over-the-counter allergy medications. Allergy shots, which desensitize one against these attacks, may also help. It's a common mistake to take an antihistamine when you have symptoms and then to stop it as soon as you get some relief. Antihistamines work best when they are taken around the clock to prevent the allergic attacks and are not as effective after the attack has already occurred. For more difficult cases, your physician may need to prescribe other more potent drugs like cortisone.

If you have persistent problems with allergic reactions and can't seem to reduce the trigger mechanisms with the above-mentioned suggestions, it's important to see your physician or allergist for further treatment.

HEADACHES

THOUGH PAINFUL, MOST AREN'T SERIOUS

Headaches come in many varieties and nearly everyone gets them at some time or other. Yet they remain mysterious, and scientists are still groping for the exact cause of the head pain.

The brain itself feels no pain. It simply interprets signals from the nearby muscles and blood vessels of the head, as well as from the membrane covering the brain. Generally, pain occurs if the nerves near the brain are being pressed upon, or if the blood vessels are either widening or narrowing.

Only rarely are headaches caused by serious illnesses such as brain tumor. Here are some of the more common, less serious types of headaches:

Tension headaches are characterized by a dull ache, especially in the back of the head, and are often triggered by stress. This stress causes the muscles of the back of the head and neck to contract for prolonged periods of time, which tightens the pressure on the nerves and tissues, as well as the nearby blood vessels. Over-the-counter pain relievers will usually help. Behavior modification and relaxation will also be necessary if the headaches become frequent and unremitting.

Migraine headaches typically affect one side of the head. Initially the pain concentrates in an area about the size of a fingertip but eventually spreads out to include half of the head. This is often accompanied by irritability, dizziness, and sometimes vomiting and sweating. There are many medications available for migraine and preventive medications often are given to those who have attacks more frequently than every two months. More commonly, treatments are prescribed to stop the migraine at its onset. Several drugs are available that can block a migraine when they are taken at the first symptoms. You need to see your physician for a prescription.

Cluster headaches come in groups of painful bouts that can only be described as excruciating. This intense pain strikes without warning on one side of the head, normally localizing around one eye. That eye might also become somewhat bloodshot. Cluster headaches are often accompanied by a teary eye and a runny nose on the same side of the face. Sometimes the pain also radiates around the face. After each series of pains, there is a headache-free period that can last up to several years. The typical cluster headache victim is a male 20 to 50 years old. Researchers speculate that cluster victims may have an abnormality of the small branches of blood vessels in the forehead which can be affected in some way by a substance in the body called histamine (cluster headaches and histamine headaches are the same thing). Stress, alcohol, and heavy smoking appear to trigger cluster headaches. Various drugs have also been tried with only uneven success. You will need to see your physician for a prescription.

Most headaches fall within the tension category and respond well to over-the-counter medication. However, if a headache persists it's important to see your physician. With proper diagnosis and treatment nearly all headaches can be relieved.

SOME UNSUSPECTED SOURCES OF HEADACHE PAIN

Some headaches can be tracked to a very specific source. Here are some unusual triggers of headache pain:

- *Chewing gum*: The relentless grinding tires the muscles around the jaw and may cause pain at the front and sides of the head.
- *Ice Cream*: Sudden cooling of the roof of the mouth causes two nerves and the tissues in that area to hurry pain signals to the brain.
- *Salt*: Too much salt can bring on migraine headaches, often hours after eating it.
- *Carbon monoxide*: Believe it or not, after a night's sleep with your head under the covers carbon monoxide can build up, cutting down on your oxygen supply and giving you a headache. Keep your head out in the open!
- *Sun*: Too much time in the sun dehydrates your body, depleting the fluids around the brain and spinal column. This causes the blood vessels to rub against these surrounding tissues and their nerves and can cause pain.
- *Mobile homes and residential construction*: The chemical formaldehyde is sometimes used in the manufacture of particle board used for mobile home floors and walls. It is also found in plywood and other building materials. A high level of formaldehyde in the air can cause headaches.
- *Overexertion*: During strenuous exercise, small blood vessels may not be able to expand fast enough to accommodate the increased blood flow. Pressure from backed up blood can build up the arteries, stretching the walls and causing a headache.
- *Spiked heels*: Wearing high heels can tense back muscles. This tension can spread up into the head and neck bringing on headaches.

Thinking about possible headache triggers in your life might help you solve your own headache problem. If the headaches are persistent, then you will need to see your physician.

HEART ATTACK—WHAT IT REALLY IS

MYOCARDIAL INFARCTION; CORONARY THROMBOSIS

There are a lot of confusing terms used to signify heart attack, and sometimes it's difficult to understand what it really is. Coronary thrombosis, myocardial infarction, and heart attack all mean basically the same thing. A stroke, however, refers to a blood clot to the brain (not the heart) and is an entirely different problem.

Essentially, as the small arteries that feed the heart begin to clog up with cholesterol, the blood flow through them is reduced. Blood carries oxygen and when the heart doesn't get enough oxygen, because of the reduced blood flow, chest pain begins to develop. These chest pains, especially those that occur with exertion, are called "angina." Angina pains normally last for about five or 15 minutes. They are usually relieved by rest and/ or taking nitroglycerin under the tongue.

When the flow through the coronary arteries becomes totally blocked, then the pain begins to last longer (anywhere from 30 minutes to three hours). This total lack of flow causes that part of the heart to die and form scar tissue. This, then, is called a heart attack because it leaves a permanent scar. Often, a small blood clot is the final culprit that closes off this narrowed vessel. In summary, angina pain represents a partial or temporary closure of the blood vessels to the heart and acts as a warning pain; total closure leads to a heart attack and permanent damage.

If you do get warning signs of angina, it's important to see your doctor or go to your local hospital. If the chest discomfort lasts up to 30 minutes or more, it may be the onset of a heart attack, and prompt attention can be lifesaving. With medical attention within three hours of the onset of pain, the clot that seals off a blood vessel can sometimes be dissolved—and the heart attack stopped—using new dissolving agents.

HEARTBURN

LOWER ESOPHAGUS OFTEN IS THE CAUSE

Heartburn pain, which has the stomach as its cause, is an uncomfortable but rarely serious condition that occurs when the digestive acids that are normally in the stomach back up into the esophagus, or food-tube. This backwash, or reflux, irritates the lining of the esophagus and produces the familiar heartburn sensation. This may also be accompanied by a bitter taste in the mouth called "water brash." Heartburn can also be accompanied by bloating of the abdomen, nausea, and even vomiting.

For many years, physicians thought that a hiatal hernia was the only cause of heartburn; we now know that the true culprit is the lower esophageal sphincter (LES). This is a muscular ring-type valve that normally keeps the connection between the esophagus and stomach closed (except after swallowing), thereby preventing acid from coming back up into the esophagus. If the valve is weak or inappropriately relaxed, it leaves a small opening through which digestive juices can percolate up into the esophagus and cause what physicians refer to as "reflux."

The best way to treat reflux or heartburn is to avoid certain foods that relax that LES sphincter muscle. These include fatty or spicy foods, chocolate, peppermint, coffee (including decaffeinated), tobacco, and alcohol. Being overweight, or wearing tight fitting clothing can also aggravate the problem. If you are afflicted with this malady, try to eat small meals more frequently and don't lie down for at least 45 minutes after you have eaten.

Prevention, as discussed above, is the best way to avoid heartburn. If it occurs in spite of these measure, antacids might provide some short-term relief. If heartburn becomes a persistent problem, your physician can offer prescription medications.

Some "heartburn" is not from the stomach but may actually come from the heart, and might indicate a more serious cardiac condition. This is especially true if the "heartburn" pain occurs with exertion rather than after eating, or if it doesn't respond to the simple measures described above, such as antacids. If in doubt, see your doctor.

HEART MURMURS

ARE THEY ALWAYS SERIOUS?

As blood flows through the valves of the heart, it creates a certain amount of turbulence or noise that can be heard with a stethoscope. If the valves are thickened or abnormal, then more turbulence, and thus more noise (a loud murmur), can be heard. Think of the sound made by a rapidly flowing stream; if a large rock is placed in the middle of the stream, the turbulence increases, and so does the noise level.

Some heart murmurs are really no problem at all. These "innocent murmurs" simply reflect the fact that the heart is beating strongly and the blood is creating a soft sound as it flows through normal valves. The only way to tell whether a murmur is innocent or abnormal is to have your physician listen to it carefully. The physician can detect certain signs of abnormality that will tell whether you have to worry about this particular murmur or not.

If you do have a heart murmur, there are some precautions to keep in mind. During any surgery or dental procedures some bacteria, or germs, may get into the blood stream. Normally, these are eliminated by the body. However, in a person with an abnormal valve, these germs seem to attach onto the valve before they can be eliminated and can cause some infection and can even destroy the valve. If you have an abnormal heart murmur, you

48

must take antibiotics shortly before, during, and after any dental or surgical procedure. This would include even a dental cleaning of your teeth. Consult your physician about this, and be sure to tell your dentist that you have a heart murmur before any procedures are done.

HEAT STROKE

MUSCLE CRAMPS CAN BE A WARNING

It's often difficult to exercise outside during hot summer days. The body has a hard time regulating its temperature when the weather is both hot and humid. The most important way to get rid of heat during exercise is through evaporation of sweat. But when the relative humidity increases significantly, less sweat is able to evaporate because there's already too much water in the air. Heavy clothing also decreases evaporation of sweat. Some medications, such as antihistamines, also may impair sweating. All this will lead to a buildup of heat in the body.

Warning signs of impending heat injury include a rise in body temperature, headache, a chilly feeling, muscle cramps, unsteady gait, and sometimes a change in mental alertness. A mild form, with body temperature not over 103 degrees F, can be treated by giving fluids, sprinkling water over the person, and fanning to enhance evaporation. Applying ice packs to the neck, abdomen, and under the arms is also useful.

Heat fatigue is the first sign of heat-related illness; you begin to feel tired and run down. It's important at this point to avoid strenuous activity and to drink plenty of fluids (but not alcohol, since this increases fluid loss).

Heat exhaustion is the next stage, and occurs when the body loses too much fluid from sweating. Victims have headaches and become nauseated. The blood pressure begins to drop. At this point it's important to cool the body immediately and to administer fluids. Getting out of the sun and into the shade will help.

Heat syncope is loss of consciousness due to lack of body fluid. This is very serious, and the patient needs to be taken to a hospital immediately. Rapid cooling and intravenous fluids will probably be necessary.

Heat stroke is the most serious form of heat illness. The body temperature can go as high as 106 degrees F. The victim can even go into a coma and, in some cases, die.

The secret to prevention is simply drinking enough water both before and during exercise. There are other fluids on the market, but water seems to be the best. Not that much sodium or potassium is lost when you sweat; it is primarily water loss. If you're planning some vigorous exercise in hot weather, it's important to increase your fluid intake, even up to two days before. Taking to 6 ounces of water about 15 minutes before beginning a race or a period of exertion and drinking about 4 ounces of water every three to four miles or periodically throughout the exertion will help. Salt tablets are not really necessary since salt lost during sweating can usually be replaced with a normal diet. Only those with prolonged exposure to heat and sweating, such as construction workers out on the road, football players, long-distance runners, and members of a marching band, need to consider taking salt tablets, and then only with the advice of a doctor.

So be careful in hot, humid weather. As soon as you start to feel tired or nauseated, or get muscle cramps, slow down your activity and get plenty of fluids. The elderly and those with health problems who are on medication (which may affect the body's heat regulation and sweating mechanisms) need to be especially cautious.

HOLIDAY DRINKING

HOW MUCH IS TOO MUCH?

I am not recommending that you drink at all, but if you do include alcohol in your holiday celebrations, remember your liver can only handle about an ounce (shot) to an ounce and a half of alcohol per hour. This is equivalent to one and a half mixed drinks, two bottles of beer, or an one 8- ounce glass of wine per hour. Anything over that begins to accumulate and cause undesirable effects. Check the following chart for more specific information based on body weight and number of drinks per hour.

Here are some tips to help you practice moderation:

- Dilute your drinks with water or ice cubes.
- Choose fruit juices as mixers rather than carbonated soft drinks. Fruit juice slows alcohol absorption and accelerates alcohol metabolism.
- Beware of the double jeopardy drinks like martinis and Manhattans that are just booze on top of booze.

KNOW YOUR LIMIT

NUMBER OF DRINKS IN ONE HOUR
APPROXIMATE BLOOD ALCOHOL CONTENT (BAC)

DRINKS	BODY WEIGHT IN POUNDS								
	100	120	140	160	180	200	220	240	
1	.04	.03	.03	.02	.02	.02	.02	.02	Reasonable
2	.08	.06	.05	.05	.04	.04	.03	.03	
3	.11	.09	.08	.07	.06	.06	.05	.05	
4	.15	.12	.11	.09	.08	.08	.07	.06	Unsafe
5	.19	.16	.13	.12	.11	.09	.09	.08	
6	.23	.19	.16	.14	.13	.11	.10	.09	
7	.26	.22	.19	.16	.15	.13	.12	.11	
8	.30	.25	.21	.19	.17	.15	.14	.13	Illegal
9	.34	.28	.24	.21	.19	.17	.15	.14	
10	.38	.31	.27	.23	.21	.19	.17	.16	

One drink = 1 oz. of 100 proof liquor or one 12-oz. beer

Subtract .01% for each hour of drinking

THE OHIO DEPARTMENT OF HIGHWAY SAFETY

51

HUMAN IMMUNODEFICIENCY VIRUS—AIDS

AN OUTLINE OF CURRENT THOUGHT

Acquired Immune Deficiency Syndrome (AIDS) is often in the news, and I thought an outline explanation of the various stages of AIDS would be useful for your understanding.

In *Stage I* there are no symptoms, though the HTLV-3 antibody titer is positive. This is a blood test that helps confirm that exposure to this particular virus has occurred. Occasionally, this blood test shows a "false positive" (it doesn't tell the truth) and further blood testing is needed to confirm it. Confirmatory tests are often recommended in order to be absolutely sure of the diagnosis.

Stage II is called the AIDS related complex (ARC) syndrome. In this case there is again a positive antibody titer, but now symptoms develop including enlargement of the lymph nodes, weight loss, gastrointestinal symptoms such as nausea and vomiting, poor appetite, fatigue, and a chronic ill feeling.

Stage III is the *disease* stage of AIDS (full-blown syndrome). Here the body's defenses are quite reduced and life-threatening infections are the primary problem. The body's immune system, which fights off infection, is not functioning. Even the germs that are normally present in the body and usually kept in check by the body's defense system now are able to cause problems (opportunistic infection). This leads to conditions of unusual pneumonias (pneumocystis carinii pneumonia), fungus infections, tuberculous-type infections, unusual skin abnormalities called Kaposi's sarcoma, and an infection caused by a germ called cytomegalovirus. These infections keep recurring and are very resistant to treatment. Victims at this stage average about 250 days in the hospital over one year's time. The outlook is extremely poor with almost 100 percent death in two years.

As of this writing there is still no cure for AIDS, although AZT shows some promise. It is still contracted primarily through homosexual contact (occasionally from heterosexual contact), blood transfusions, and contaminated needles in drug abuse.

THE SILENT KILLER

High blood pressure, or hypertension, is called the silent killer—and for good reason. Most people are unaware that they even have it until it is too late. It's important for all of us to know what our blood pressure is and what factors can predispose us to this disease.

These are some predisposing factors:

- *Age*. The older you get the more likely you are to have high blood pressure.
- *Race*. While one out of every four people in the U.S. population as a whole has high blood pressure, the incidence is one out of every three in African-Americans.
- *Heredity*. High blood pressure appears to run in some families.
- *Sex*. Men are more likely than women to have hypertension.

Other factors, which are controllable, aggravate hypertension. They include excessive sodium (salt) and alcohol consumption, oral contraceptives, lack of exercise, and obesity. Individuals who weigh 20 percent or more than they should are more likely to develop high blood pressure.

And then there are some myths about hypertension. One is that loss of excess weight alone will cure high blood pressure. While weight reduction is often necessary, and it might be accompanied by reduction in pressure, some continued treatment is still required in many cases.

Another myth is that a person with hypertension is tense or anxious. Wrong. You do not have to be nervous, tense, or jumpy to develop high blood pressure.

Have your blood pressure checked annually. It is probably the easiest and most important thing you can do to increase your longevity.

IMMUNIZATIONS FOR ADULTS

THEY'RE NOT JUST FOR KIDS

Parents often schedule physical examinations and immunizations for their children at the beginning of the school year. That's a good time to remember that adults need to be immunized as well. Flu shots, pneumonia shots, and hepatitis B vaccines are generally underused in adults. Remember to keep adequate records of whatever shots you have had. The following are guidelines for six vaccines that are recommended for routine use:

DPT: This stands for Diptheria, Pertussis (whooping cough) and Tetanus. After the primary immunization in childhood, adults should receive tetanus and diptheria boosters about every 10 years. The pertussis portion is used for children less than seven years old and is not recommended for routine use in adults.

Measles: Measles is becoming more common and can be more severe in young adults than in children. It is currently recommended that anyone born after 1956 who did not receive live measles vaccine after age one and has no documented history of measles infection should receive a single dose of measles vaccine. If you are uncertain about a past history of measles, a blood test can determine if you've had the infection previously. People born in 1956 or before are probably immune. Persons vaccinated between 1963 and 1967 with inactivated measles vaccine should probably be revaccinated to prevent severe atypical measles. You should discuss this with your physician.

Rubella: The objective of immunizing adults against rubella (German measles) is to prevent spread of infection to the developing fetus. If the disease is contracted in early pregnancy, fetal infection can occur in 80 percent of cases. Therefore, routine immunization of adults is recommended, particularly for previously unimmunized women of child-bearing age and for employees of pediatric or obstetric health care facilities who don't have blood tests showing evidence of previous immunity to German measles. This blood test can be obtained through your doctor.

Influenza: Each fall between September and November you should consider getting a flu shot. It markedly reduces the complications and death rate due to influenza, especially in the elderly. Annual immunization is recommended for those with any type of chronic medical problems, such as heart or lung disease, and for everyone over 65 years of age. Adverse reactions or side effects to this vaccine have been very infrequent in the last few years.

Pneumonia vaccine: This protects you from about 90 percent of the types of pneumonia currently active in this country. Anyone with chronic medical problems, such as heart or lung disease, and especially those over 65 years of age should receive this injection. It is about 60 to 75 percent effective in most people, and one dose appears to protect you for life.

Hepatitis B vaccine: Hepatitis B, or serum hepatitis, is associated with an inflammation of the liver. It is commonly found in intravenous drug abusers, homosexuals, and among household members and sexual partners of people who have hepatitis. It can also occur in dialysis patients and health care workers. All of these people should receive this vaccine. The new way of producing this vaccine seems to avoid any problem with AIDS, and even pregnancy is not a contraindication.

INSOMNIA

HOW TO AVOID THOSE LONG, LONELY NIGHTS

For some people, the long, frustrating nights of insomnia can be devastating. I offer the following suggestions to help prevent insomnia:

- Decrease your activity before going to bed. Relax and try to reduce your tension level.
- Don't drink alcohol or caffeinated beverages before retiring. Some over-the-counter medications have caffeine in them; check the ingredients.

- Read a book until your eyes get very heavy.
- Focus on an object on the ceiling and try to "move it" with your eyes. This is fatiguing for your eyes and might help to promote sleep.
- Don't fight it! You can't force sleep; you simply have to relax and let it happen.
- Have some milk or bananas. They contain a substance called tryptophane which seems to help promote relaxation and sleep.
- Some prescription medications (antihistamines, heart, and lung pills) can affect the amount of dreaming that you do and can lead to a restless sleep. You should discuss this with your physician.
- While sleeping pills can be used as a last resort, you should see your physician for the one that would be best for you. Some sleeping pills send you into such a deep sleep that they suppress the amount that you dream, which will prevent you from feeling well-rested in the morning. You need to find one that allows a more natural sleep and is not habit-forming. If you must take sleeping pills regularly, try to take them just three out of four weeks in any one month in order to have at least one week off to allow your body to readjust.

IRRITABLE BOWEL SYNDROME

IT ISN'T NECESSARILY COLITIS

Irritable bowel syndrome (IBS) is often confused with colitis (inflammation of the colon). Although IBS is a very common disorder, it is one that many people know little about.

Irritable bowel syndrome is characterized by harsh, spasmodic contractions of the bowel usually 30 to 45 minutes after eating. This is felt as discomfort in the lower left portion of the abdomen. Diarrhea usually follows and then symptoms disappear. At other times, these erratic contractions actually delay emptying of the bowel, causing some constipation.

The major cause of irritable bowel syndrome is a person's reaction to emotional stress. The symptoms might not always coincide exactly with the stress; they might even occur after the crisis has passed. Another cause of the disorder is sensitivity to certain foods, beverages, and drugs. The severity of the symptoms varies from person to person and from one episode to another. People from age 15 to 45 are the most susceptible.

What can be done? Eat at regularly scheduled times and don't skip meals. Avoid foods that don't agree with your system, and don't overeat. Also, remember to eat slowly and try to relax while you are eating. Your doctor may also suggest adding bran or fiber to your diet. Take advantage of the bowel's tendency to empty after each meal, especially after breakfast. And try to get 30 to 45 minutes of physical activity every day, even if it's just walking around the block a few times.

If the problem persists or becomes more severe, your doctor might want to prescribe medication. It's important to discuss this condition with your doctor in order to rule out colitis or bowel tumors (See *Colitis,* page 23).

THE USE OF LASERS IN MEDICINE

THE CUTTING EDGE OF SURGERY

The word laser is an acronym for *l*ight *a*mplification by *s*timulated *e*mission of *r*adiation. A laser is an instrument that produces an intense, highly focused beam of light that is so powerful it can drill a hole in a diamond, yet so accurate it can be aimed through the pupil of a human eye to weld a detached retina back in place.

Lasers were first and most commonly used in ophthamology for diseases of the eye. They were used to repair retinal tears and to fix retinal complications of diabetes. The newer lasers allow the ophthalmologist to treat both the back of the eye (the retina) and the front of the eye. Often the entire operative procedure can be done on an outpatient basis. Even glaucoma, an increase in the fluid pressure of the eye, can be treated with lasers.

Lasers have many advantages in neurosurgery since they allow precise cutting of tumors, with good evaporation near the edge of the cut, and less bleeding. They even sterilize as they cut.

Lasers have been used to eliminate blockages of the breathing tubes that can occur secondary to tumors. They can also be used to coagulate blood vessels that may bleed inside of these breathing tubes.

Lasers have been successful in opening up blockages in the arteries of the legs. Although it is still not a proven treatment at the time of this writing, lasers may ultimately open up blocked arteries around the heart.

Lasers can be an advantage in surgery since they can reduce the risk, time involved, and bleeding associated with surgery. However, effective surgery doesn't require use of a laser to make an incision. You can discuss with your doctor whether using a laser would represent a real gain in your case.

LEGIONNAIRE'S DISEASE

IT'S STILL AROUND AND PROBABLY COMMON

Do you remember all the news headlines about the Legionnaire's disease epidemic in Philadelphia in 1976? Legionnaire's disease is a form of pneumonia that has probably been around for a long time and occurs much more often than we formerly thought.

In an epidemic situation it affects a group of people who are essentially fit and young to middle-aged, who will all become infected at the same time. This usually occurs after exposure to dust or contaminated water containing the bacterium *Legionella pneumophila*. After an incubation period of 24 to 36 hours, victims usually come down with fever, headache, aching pain in the muscles, dry cough, chest pain, and sometimes nausea and diarrhea.

More sporadic and individual cases involve people whose resistance to infection has become reduced, or who are exposed to a greater than usual concentration of this germ. They always have a more dramatic illness with more severe chills and fever, muscle aches, heavy sweating, mental confusion, slurred speech, and in some cases a "galloping" form of pneumonia that destroys lung tissue and can lead to death. The factors that depress immunity and predispose people to this more severe form include alcoholism, dialysis, diabetes, heart trouble, heavy smoking, rheumatoid arthritis and certain medications like cortisone drugs.

We can't totally avoid the bacteria since they are abundantly present in the air or in contaminated water. Luckily, antibiotic treatment with erythromycin or tetracycline quickly brings the disease under control and prevents complications and fatalities if the medication is started early enough.

LONGEVITY

HOW TO LIVE TO BE 100

Studies of people who have lived to be over 100 years old (primarily in the Soviet Union) provide some tips on how to live to a ripe old age. If you detect a bit of humor in some of these suggestions—well, humor is one of the keys to longevity.

- •. Be married.
- • Stay in one geographic location.
- • Do some physical activity every day.
- • Go to bed no later than 8 or 9 p.m. and sleep up to 10 hours per day.
- • Take long walks.
- • Eat in moderation. Concentrate on vegetables, salads and fruits. Cover your foods with spicy sauces made from red and black pepper. Use honey and not sugar for the sweetener.
- • Drink a bit of homemade wine before meals.
- • Avoid smoking.
- • Eat three to four times a day at specific times and always slightly undereat, with lunch as your main meal.
- • Limit sexual activity. (Sorry!)

Now don't despair just because you can's eat spicy foods or follow some of the other suggestions. It doesn't mean that you can't incorporate some of these suggestions into your daily life. If you eat right, stay fit, and enjoy the nontoxic good things in life, you will have a good chance of being around a long time.

LUNCH AND THE MID-AFTERNOON SLUMP

CAN YOU AVOID IT?

What you eat for lunch does have some effect on how you will feel in the afternoon. But no matter what you eat, chances are good that you will still have a mid-day slump. This slump is in part a normal response to a daily dip in the body temperature. You can reduce the impact of that drop in temperature, and the corresponding slump, by watching what you eat for lunch. Studies indicate that reaction times and intellectual skills are much better after eating turkey (protein) than after eating a high-carbohydrate lunch. The adverse effects of carbohydrates last for about three hours after you eat!

How much you eat is also significant. Another study found that people make more mistakes on tests after eating a heavy meal of 1,000 calories than after a light lunch of 300 calories. But skipping lunch is taking it too far. Most studies show that people perform even worse on an empty stomach. In addition, changes in normal routine, such as eating more or less than usual, also increases errors.

So check out the lunch menu for a low-calorie, high-protein lunch. It will help you survive that mid-afternoon slump.

WHO NEEDS THEM? ARE THEY SAFE?

When former First Lady Nancy Reagan developed breast cancer, the news stories drew national attention to the problem. At that time, the medical report on Mrs. Reagan indicated that on a routine mammogram her doctors found a 7mm tumor (very small) in her breast. The fact that she had a mammogram gets the credit for this discovery since this size tumor would be very difficult to feel on examination.

Breast cancer is the number one killer in women. Widespread awareness of the use of mammograms is vital. Currently, the American Cancer Society recommends all women over 50 undergo routine breast x-rays every year to look for tumors. They recommend getting a baseline mammogram between the ages of 35 and 39 so that later x-rays can be compared to it. In addition, the Cancer Society says that all women over 20 should examine their breasts each month for lumps or other changes, and they should be examined by a physician every three years. After age 40, the exam by the physician should be yearly.

Mammography is nothing more than a low radiation x-ray that allows a doctor to detect very small tumors in the breast *before they can be felt.* There is essentially no radiation danger from this test.

I cannot emphasize enough the importance of routine breast examinations and mammography. The long-term survival rate for breast cancer is nearly 100 percent if it is caught before it invades other tissue.

MEGAVITAMINS

ARE THEY WORTH IT? ARE THEY HARMFUL?

Taking vitamin supplements is a popular national pastime. Three out of four Americans believe that taking extra vitamins will give them more pep no matter how adequate their diets are. Many believe that high-dose vitamins will prevent arthritis, cancer, even the common cold. Unfortunately, each year there are nearly 4,000 cases of vitamin poisoning; 80 percent of these are in children.

Taking recommended doses of vitamins is a reasonable thing to do. The "megadose" problem occurs in people who take at least 10 times more than the recommended daily allowance. Some physicians consider that these excessive amounts act more like drugs than they do as nutrients.

The following are some examples of vitamins and the problems they can cause:

- *B vitamins*: These are popular and supposedly calm nerves and act as a mood boosters. The most common side effect is liver damage if taken in excess of 50 mg per day.
- *Vitamin C*: This is supposed to protect one from everything from colds to cancer. Using 500 to 1,000 mg per day is probably not going to cause any trouble. With more than that, susceptible individuals risk some side effects such as nausea, abdominal cramps, diarrhea, and kidney stones. In addition, vitamin C interferes with the test for blood in the stool. Vitamin C probably does help to reduce the severity of colds, but it is important not to overdo this one.
- *Vitamin A*: This is advertised as an anti-infection factor and as being good for the skin. A good supplement will contain about 10,000 IU. However, excessive doses taken for a long time can cause skin disease, hair loss, headache, diarrhea, blurred vision, as well as liver, kidney, and bone damage. Be careful with this one!

- *Vitamin D*: Vitamin D is an important vitamin because it facilitates calcium absorption in the intestine. However, it is also one of the most toxic of the so-called fat-soluble vitamins and, when taken in excessive amounts, can cause significantly elevated calcium levels in the body. This extra calcium can then be deposited in tissues or form kidney stones, which could result in irreversible kidney damage.
- *Vitamin E*: This is advertised to lower cholesterol and improve circulation. Excessive doses of this can cause blurred vision, depression and fatigue, headaches, and abnormalities of blood clotting leading to possible bleeding. Don't take this if you're on a blood thinner!

Now I am not against vitamin therapy. It is beneficial in many cases. But you must be careful if you are going to take excessive doses, and you should probably consult your physician before you attempt this. You can usually get enough vitamins by eating a balanced diet. If you think you need extra, then at least discuss the vitamin supplement program with your doctor.

MENINGITIS

WHAT SHOULD YOU DO IF YOU'RE EXPOSED?

Meningitis is a dreaded disease that causes infection and swelling of the spinal cord and brain and sometimes death.

Meningitis is caught in much the same way that we catch a cold, from exposure to someone who has the disease. Some people are also "carriers" of the meningitis germ who can pass the disease to others without getting sick themselves. It all depends on your body's ability to fight it off.

The symptoms of meningitis include high fever, severe headache, nausea, vomiting, and a personality change, especially in children. With proper attention this severe illness can be cured.

Meningitis can be caused by either a virus or bacteria. For a bacterial infection, antibiotics are necessary and must be given promptly. Sometimes the only way of determining whether the cause is bacterial or viral is to use a needle to take a small sample of the spinal fluid (spinal tap). With a viral infection some treatments are available. However, rest, fluids, and "tincture of time" allow most people to recover spontaneously.

If you are exposed to anyone with meningitis, it is first necessary to find out whether it is bacterial or viral. If it is viral, there is really no good preventive treatment, so you must just wait and see. If it's bacterial, any family members or intimate contacts need to be given antibiotics right away. It is important to talk to your doctor as soon as you find out you have been exposed to bacterial meningitis.

MITRAL VALVE PROLAPSE

IT MIMICS HEART ATTACK, BUT IS RELATIVELY BENIGN

Perhaps you know of someone who has a cardiac condition called "prolapse" of the mitral valve. It affects 10 to 15 percent of females and a significant proportion of males as well. In this condition the mitral valve inside the heart is too long for the size of the heart and tends to flop back and forth with each beat of the heart. For reasons not completely understood, this flopping causes irritability of the heart, resulting in extra beats or palpitations, along with chest pain and occasional lightheadedness and dizziness. Fatigue may also be a problem.

Although the tendency for this condition is present from birth, it doesn't start causing trouble until somewhere in the teens, twentie,s or thirties. Unfortunately, the symptoms that it causes can be frightening and often mimic more severe forms of heart disease. Listening carefully to the heart with a stethoscope may reveal a murmur and a "click." The condition can be fairly easily diagnosed through a painless test called an echocardiogram, which takes a sonar picture of the heart. Although reassurance is often sufficient, medications are occasionally necessary to control the symptoms. The outlook for those with mitral valve prolapse is quite good since it does not lead to a heart attack nor does it usually require any significant change in lifestyle. It has been suggested, however, that antibiotics should be taken prior to any dental or surgical work, since germs that get into the bloodstream during these procedures might cause an infection on this valve.

On very rare occasions the mitral valve might have to be surgically replaced because of intractable pain or leakage problems.

If you have any of these symptoms of chest pain, palpitations, or dizziness, you should see your physician to find out if you have a prolapse of the mitral valve. If you do, it will ease your mind to know that this condition usually is not serious and does not lead to heart attacks.

MONONUCLEOSIS

A CAUSE OF CHRONIC FATIGUE SYNDROME?

Mononucleosis is a common problem in people 15 to 25 years old. We now know that a virus called the Epstein-Barr (EB) virus is the most frequent cause of this disease. "Mono" is associated with a sore throat, fever, swollen lymph glands and significant weakness and tiredness. It often strikes in early spring or fall and generally gets better by itself in 2 to 4 weeks without treatment other than rest. However, the spleen can become very large and fragile and can be ruptured with only minor trauma. This is why mononucleosis victims must avoid contact sports for several months even after they have recovered.

Mononucleosis is caught in the same way as a cold, and it really has nothing specific to do with kissing, though it has been called the "kissing disease." Being exposed, in a close fashion, to someone who has mononucleosis is the easiest way to get it, especially if you happen to be run down at the time.

Unfortunately, there is new evidence that chronic mononucleosis syndrome can occur when this EB virus lingers in the body for a long time (chronic fatigue syndrome, "yuppie" disease). Patients have intermittent sore throats, fever, fatigue, and sometimes a feeling of gloom. They might not even be aware that they had mononucleosis in the first place.

Blood tests can show the presence of a persistently high concentration of the EB virus which is responsible for the disease. It is not known why the body can't rid itself of the EB virus, and extra rest seems to be the only way to cope with these symptoms. After several months to a year most people begin to feel better. In a few cases the illness may last longer.

In 20- to 30-year-old patients who develop vague fatigue, and seem to have lost interest in work or school, physicians are now suggesting that one of the first things to test for is the chronic fatigue syndrome and the EB virus.

MOTION SICKNESS

PREVENTION IS THE ONLY TREATMENT

No matter what the form of transportation, motion sickness can make getting from here to there a very uncomfortable business. How can you prevent it?

- Alcoholic beverages are certainly to be avoided.
- "Keep your eyes on the horizon" is a time-honored suggestion.
- Don't read in the car.
- Sit in the front of the bus away from the "rock and roll" motion of the back.
- Good ventilation while riding, including using the air conditioner, can help to reduce the symptoms.
- Some motion sickness pills are available over-the-counter.
- One simple remedy is to take 2 to 3 ginger root capsules a half hour before traveling. The advantage of this remedy is that it

is natural and has very few side effects. The capsules are sold at some drugstores and health food stores.

- One of the newer and more effective preventive treatments is a Scopolamine patch. It's a small disc that is put behind your ear two to 12 hours prior to the expected motion discomfort. It works for about 72 hours. It does have some side effects, including dry mouth, drowsiness, and blurred vision. It is not recommended for children or the elderly, nor for anyone with liver or kidney problems, stomach blockage, bladder trouble, or glaucoma. You will need to see your doctor to obtain this prescription treatment.

NIGHTTIME MUSCLE CRAMPS

TIPS TO AVOID THIS BEDTIME ANNOYANCE

No one really knows what causes muscle cramps at night, but they can be a nightmare for those who suffer from them. To help prevent them while you are in bed, place your foot in a neutral position, bent neither up nor down. For example, if you sleep on your back, keep the covers loose so your feet are not bent one way or the other. If you sleep on your stomach, allow your feet to extend over the edge of the mattress maintaining them in a neutral position.

The quickest way to get relief from a cramped muscle is to flex it. Stand up and lean forward with your hands against the wall for support. Or grasp hold of your toes and pull the foot towards you in a flexed position. If you feel a knot in the muscle, massaging the area will often help.

Dr. Donald Cooper, a former U.S. Olympic team doctor, found that something called the "acupinch" works quite well. Take a firm hold of your upper lip just below the nose with your thumb and index finger (both of them on the outside of the upper lip) and pinch for 20 to 30 seconds. This works about 80 percent of the time.

If you suffer from frequent muscle cramps you might be deficient in calcium. Increase your intake of calcium-rich foods like yogurt, cheese, and green vegetables. There are prescription medications (quinine preparations) that can be taken at bedtime. If the cramps are not relieved by theses simple measures, or if they begin to occur during the daytime, consult your physician. Circulation problems or nerve injuries could be at fault.

MUSHROOM POISONING

LEAVE MUSHROOMING TO THE EXPERTS

Wild mushroom enthusiasts find a plentiful harvest in late summer and early fall. There are thousands of species of wild mushrooms. As many as 100 mushroom species are poisonous. The toxic and nontoxic species often grow in the same places and often resemble each other. Even a trained person might have difficulty distinguishing the edible from the poisonous.

Symptoms of mushroom poisoning include nausea, vomiting, abdominal pain, and diarrhea. Excessive perspiration and salivation as well as disturbed vision can also occur. The most common types of mushroom poisoning usually begin to produce symptoms six to 12 hours after eating. However, for more toxic types, the onset can be as soon as 30 minutes.

Treatment of mushroom poisoning depends on the type of toxin, but all alert victims should be given 2 teaspoons of syrup of ipecac to induce vomiting if it has not already occurred. After the vomiting has stopped, drinking a slurry of activated charcoal in water, which can be purchased at a pharmacy and kept at home, can help to prevent the toxin in the stomach from being absorbed. If you don't have activated charcoal, use the scrapings from burnt toast (enough to provide two teaspoonsful of charred material).

Most types of mushroom poisoning resolve spontaneously with no problems, but certain types can be fatal. Remember to induce vomiting, give activated charcoal, and then call the poison control center and your physician for further information. If you end up going to the hospital, bring along some of the mushrooms that you think may have been eaten, to aid in identification.

MYTHS ABOUT HEART DISEASE

THERE IS NO MAGIC WAND

These are some cherished myths about one's likelihood of developing heart trouble:

• **None of my relatives died of heart disease so I probably won't either.** Although there is an important hereditary component to heart trouble, it is simply one of the many risk factors. If heredity were a major factor in heart disease, then the Japanese, who seem to be genetically protected by virtue of their low cardiovascular death rate, should maintain that advantage when moving to the United States. But this is not the case. When these immigrants adopt our lifestyle, they also adopt our way of death!

• **My cholesterol level is normal so I am safe.** Americans in general have relatively high cholesterol levels compared to people in other countries. The new guidelines suggest that you are not adequately protected unless your cholesterol level gets below 200 . Even people with normal cholesterol levels can still have heart attacks. Cholesterol is just one of the many factors in the development of heart disease.

• **Exercise will protect me.** Although aerobic exercise does have definite benefits for the cardiovascular system, and it might improve survival after a heart attack, there is really no good evidence that it actually prevents heart attacks. Exercise can lower your cholesterol and improve your circulation, and it is definitely to be recommended. But it is not 100 percent effective. Runners get heart attacks, too.

OSTEOPOROSIS

SHOULD YOU TAKE CALCIUM AND/OR HORMONES?

Osteoporosis is a thinning of the bone that occurs primarily in women after menopause and to a certain extent in men as they age. It happens more often in women because they have 30 percent less bone mass than men and can afford to lose less. As the hormones decline with age, the calcium in the bones also begins to decrease, and the bones become weak and brittle. Then there is danger of fractures of the spine and hips.

Recent studies suggest that after menopause women should be placed on hormones in order to prevent this bone loss. It appears that both estrogen and progesterone should be taken on a daily basis (3 weeks on, 1 week off). The disadvantage and inconvenience is that if the uterus is still present there will be some monthly bleeding. It's like starting over with menstrual periods again. There is some controversy as to whether this is effective and whether the risk of possibly developing breast cancer makes it worthwhile.

Current thought suggests that increasing calcium and vitamin D in your diet, as well as adding exercise to your daily schedule, can do the job just as well. Calcium supplements can slow down bone loss, while the exercise puts some stress on the bones, which helps to promote bone growth. The exercise does not need to be of the olympic variety; even just walking two to three times per week will make a significant improvement. Posture and back exercises (see page 7) are also important.

A BOTHERSOME BEATING OF THE HEART

It startles you when it happens. Some people describe it as a "flip-flop" inside the chest. Others feel a "lump in the throat." You might think your heart has "skipped a beat."

Actually, these are extra beats that occur prematurely in the normal cycle. It's not the extra beat that you feel; it's the pause that follows it that causes the skipping sensation. So although one may feel there has been a stoppage of the heart, in reality it is simply the natural pause that occurs while the heart resets itself to its normal cycle. That pause allows extra blood to accumulate in the heart, making the next beat more forceful. This causes the flip-flop or thumping sensation inside the chest.

These premature or extra beats are usually nothing to worry about. They can come in the course of a normal day, especially if you've had a lot of caffeinated coffee or colas. Both smoking and stress definitely aggravate the condition.

Some medications contribute to it. If you have palpitations, first try to eliminate the coffee, smoking, and stress. If the palpitations persist, then it is time to make a trip to your physician's office. You can ask about any medications you're taking. And it's important to be sure that there is no underlying heart disease to account for the palpitations.

WHEN AND HOW TO TAKE PILLS

BEFORE, DURING, OR AFTER MEALS?

In spite of our best efforts and good intentions, sometimes we do get sick and have to take medication. The doctor is likely to instruct us to take the pills "with meals." But does that mean before, during, or after meals?

In general, a pill taken before eating is absorbed better and therefore works better in your system. However, certain medications that might upset the stomach, such as aspirin preparations and arthritis medications, are better taken with food. Some medications are inactivated by acidity and should not be taken with fruit juices or carbonated beverages; various antibiotics are included on this list. Other medications are made less absorbable by the calcium in milk (for example, the antibiotic tetracycline). Furthermore, milk might dissolve the coating on some pills that is intended to reduce stomach irritation (for example, enteric-coated aspirin).

In summary, most pills are better taken before meals—unless the prescription bottle says something else. If you're not sure, ask your doctor or pharmacist if fruit juice or milk are all right to use with the pills, and whether the pills need to be taken with food.

POISON IVY

IT'S MORE OF AN ALLERGY

Summertime is poison ivy time. The woods, fence lines, and even your own backyard can harbor an abundant crop of this pesky plant. It is not just direct contact with the leaves that can cause an outbreak; oils from the plant leaves can be transmitted by brushing garden tools against plants and then grasping the tools. Even burning the plants, which can create poison-filled smoke, can infect many people over a large area.

The best way to avoid poison ivy is to get to know the plants by sight. They generally have three leaves and grow as low bushes or climbing vines. They are sometimes mixed with honeysuckle and other climbers.

If you do become exposed to the poisonous plants, carefully remove your clothes and thoroughly wash all the affected areas of skin with warm water and soap. Using a sponge, apply a 50 to

70 percent alcohol solution to the area. Wearing gloves, wash your clothes in soapy water. Dry them in the sun.

Itching and redness of the skin will occur within several hours or several days after exposure. Watery blisters appearing in the affected area will confirm that you have the poison ivy infection. Although there are many over-the-counter medications to relieve the pain and itch of poison ivy, be sure to contact your physician for the best advice. If your symptoms are bad enough, he or she may want to give you a cortisone shot.

THE PROSTATE GLAND

THIS "PRESIDENTIAL DISEASE" IS COMMON AMONG ALL MEN

When President Reagan developed prostate problems, public awareness of the problem increased.

The prostate gland is a small, walnut-sized gland that sits at the base of the penis. With the aging process, this gland begins to enlarge and gradually presses against the opening of the bladder, thereby restricting the flow of urine.

The symptoms of an enlarged prostate include frequent urination, especially during the night, and difficulty in initiating the urinary stream. Bladder infections also seem to occur more frequently, and bleeding can be a problem.

As the urine flow becomes more and more obstructed, surgery of this gland has to be considered. This is typically carried out by a urologist who inserts a hollow metal tube into the urethra, or opening of the penis. The patient is anesthetized during this process. Small pieces of the prostate on the inside of the bladder are cut away to open up the bladder's passage for urine.

Most often the cause of this enlargement is simply some benign growth. If a cancerous tumor is present, the prostate will need to be removedsurgically, and some follow-up radiation treatments might also be needed.

Although prostate gland enlargement is usually not a problem until after the age of 50, every man aged 40 and over should have yearly prostate examinations in order to detect any early signs of cancer. A new blood test for prostate specific antigen can help detect prostate cancer. Ask your doctor.

PULSE RATE

WHAT'S NORMAL AT REST AND AFTER EXERCISE?

What is a normal pulse rate? For most adults around 70 beats per minute is thought to be ideal. In general, lower pulse rates are desirable since a slow resting pulse (55 to 70) indicates that the heart is working at optimum efficiency with the least energy expenditure.

The resting pulse might be higher during times of high emotional or mental strain and in high temperature situations such as in a sauna or steam room. The pulse can rise as high as 200 beats per minute during some of these situations.

A slow resting pulse is good up to a point. A resting pulse in the 50 to 60 range may represent good physical conditioning— if you have been exercising. However, if your pulse is excessively slow (less than 55), and you have not been in training, it could represent a medical problem such as an abnormality of the heart's own pacemaker. This is especially likely if symptoms of lightheadedness or passing out have occurred.

If you're starting an exercise program and want to know how high your pulse should go during exercise use the following formula:

> Subtract your *age* from *220* to get your
> *maximum pulse*. Then use 85 percent of this
> value during any strenuous exercise.

If you are just starting an exercise program talk to your doctor first about checking your blood pressure, your cholesterol, and setting some reasonable limits. This is especially true if you're over 40 and/or have a family history of heart problems.

THE RETINA OF THE EYE

YOUR DOCTOR'S WINDOW TO YOUR HEALTH

The eye is the body's only transparent organ. Your doctor routinely beams a light through your pupils to get a look at the retina at the back of the eye. The retina is a delicate multilayered area of specialized cells and blood vessels. Different spots and patches can show up here that might signal diseases of the eye or body. The blood vessels can also show evidence of diseases such as high blood pressure, cholesterol deposits, or diabetes.

RHEUMATIC FEVER IS MAKING A COMEBACK

WHEN SHOULD YOU TREAT A SORE THROAT?

In the past few years, the number of diagnosed cases of rheumatic fever has been increasing significantly in the United States.

This disorder begins as a strep infection of the throat, but it is the complication of that infection that can cause the permanent heart damage and even death associated with rheumatic fever. When a strep infection occurs, the body produces antibodies to fight off the bacteria. Some people, for reasons unknown, produce an excess of antibodies. These antibodies not only attack the strep bacteria but also the heart, joint tissue, and sometimes the brain. This is rheumatic fever. It's the body "turning on itself."

The tendency to develop rheumatic fever seems to be inherited, and it most often attacks infants to young adults (most common ages five to 15). No one knows for certain why the disorder is becoming more prevalent; perhaps because of less vigilance in obtaining throat cultures. It is most common in densely populated urban centers and crowded areas such as military barracks and closed institutions.

What we do know is that the only way to avoid rheumatic fever completely is to treat a strep infection within three days of its onset, before the body begins producing antibodies. This is usually easily accomplished with penicillin, or with alternate antibiotics for those allergic to penicillin.

If you have a sore throat for 24 hours, it is a good idea to see your doctor. Since it takes about 24 hours to get the culture results, you'll still be within the three-day time frame for effective treatment.

Anyone between 18 months and 25 years of age who has a severe sore throat accompanied by fever that does not go away should have a throat culture taken. The only way to beat rheumatic fever is to catch it early.

SHIN SPLINTS

AN EXERCISE-RELATED INJURY

Runners and aerobic dancers give their lower legs a pounding. Sometimes pain develops along the "shin bone" — the front or inner part of the leg between knee and ankle. The condition is called shin splints. Any unusual increase in walking or running, especially if you're not in condition can cause the problem. In mild cases, you feel an ache during a workout, but it doesn't necessarily stop you from exercising. In more severe cases, you might have to stop for rest periods, or even stop exercising altogether.

Shin splints are probably caused by slight tearing of the muscles of the lower leg, with some associated swelling. However they can sometimes be a symptom of the more serious problem of stress fractures, which are hairline cracks of the surface of the bone.

The following measures will help you relieve or prevent shin splints:

- Apply ice and take aspirin for temporary relief.

- Examine the surface on which you exercise; hard non-giving surfaces are especially likely to contribute to this condition.

- Look at your exercise schedule. Any recent, rapid increase in your exercise program could be the cause of shin splints; so cut back for a while.

- Examine your shoes; they should have good shock-absorbing features.

- Watch out for hills, especially downhill running. It can lead to shin splints.

If the pain persists for more than two weeks, you might have a stress fracture. Your physician might want to schedule an x-ray and will probably prescribe rest.

SIDS — SUDDEN INFANT DEATH SYNDROME

HOW TO SPOT TROUBLE SIGNS IN YOUR CHILD

There is much we need to learn about this fatal illness. Sudden infant death syndrome (SIDS) seems to strike without warning, leaving a family devastated by the unexplainable death of an apparently healthy baby.

SIDS usually affects babies less than six months old. The most common symptom is breathing difficulty. While this isn't always easy for parents to detect, medical experts have determined that there are some clear signs of trouble. If your baby turns blue at any time or has a disruptive, irregular breathing pattern or stops breathing for 10 seconds or more, it is important to see your doctor.

The cause of SIDS is still not understood. However, some babies are at higher risk for SIDS than others:

- Infants born prematurely.
- Those whose brother or sister had SIDS or a "near miss" with SIDS.
- Babies who turn blue when being fed.
- Those with any type of respiratory disease such as pneumonia or bronchitis. These breathing problems caused by these infections might be more severe for babies, since they can only breathe through their noses in early infancy.

If you are a parent of an infant, don't panic; simply take care of your baby as you normally would. If your family has a history of SIDS, or if you notice your baby having any breathing or feeding problems, then contact your doctor.

SILENT HEART ATTACKS

YOU CAN HAVE A HEART ATTACK AND NOT EVEN KNOW IT

Each year some people die from heart attacks seemingly without any warning. These are so-called "silent heart attacks," and medical experts feel that as many as 5 *million* Americans may be having them.

It is possible to have multiple, small, silent heart attacks that go unrecognized. Although these might not cause death, research shows that the effects of these silent heart attacks are cumulative. As a result, more and more scar tissue builds up in the heart.

It is very important to detect silent heart attacks early and prevent more attacks with appropriate therapy. Here is where your doctor becomes a detective. One of the ways to detect these episodes is with a 24-hour Holter monitor. This is a small recording device connected with wires to small patches placed on the chest wall. This device records each heartbeat on an electrocardiogram over a 24-hour period. The patient wears the monitor throughout the course of a normal day's activity. Computer analysis of the recorded data reveals any evidence of silent heart attacks.

Diagnosis can also be established by doing a treadmill or stress test. Even though the patient might not experience any chest discomfort ("silent heart pain") during the treadmill test, an electrocardiogram might pick up changes in heart performance that suggest blocked arteries.

Treatment can significantly modify the risk of silent heart attack. Losing weight and lowering blood pressure can help. Drug therapy might be necessary. In more severe cases, cardiac catheterization and/or coronary bypass surgery might be necessary.

Silent heart attacks not only strike without warning, they don't seem to be linked with physical activity either. If you have

79

significant risk factors for heart disease (cholesterol, smoking, strong family history), you might want to ask your doctor about being tested for this silent cardiac problem.

SIT-UPS

WILL THEY REALLY HELP REDUCE THAT ABDOMINAL BULGE?

Most people tend to gain weight in the abdomen; fat concentrates there all too easily and usually refuses to budge. It's been popular to do sit-ups in an attempt to reduce fat in the abdomen. I'm afraid I have some bad news for you; so called "spot reducing" doesn't work. In research done on college students, abdominal fat was measured both before and after doing about 5,000 sit-ups over 27 days. There was no difference in the amount of fat lost in the abdominal area compared to other sites on the body.

Moreover, sit-ups can cause lower back problems if they are not done correctly. The best method is to lie on your back with your knees bent and your toes locked under an immovable object. First raise your head until your chin touches your chest. Then gradually raise your back off the floor until you're about halfway up, and then lie back down again. This concentrates maximum muscle tension in the abdominal muscles with less stress on the lower back.

While exercising specific areas of the body might lead to firmer muscles in those areas, it is not likely to reduce fat from that part of the body. You simply have to lose weight in general, and hope that eventually it will come off the area of concern.

SNORING IS SOMETIMES THE SYMPTOM OF A DISEASE

Sleep apnea is a condition in which a person periodically stops breathing while asleep. This interrupts the sleep pattern, causing excessive daytime drowsiness. It can also reduce the oxygen content of the blood and can lead to irregularities of the heart rhythm.

There are two basic types of sleep apnea: Central sleep apnea is due to an inability of the brain to correctly signal the breathing pattern while one is asleep. The cause of this is uncertain. Obstructive sleep apnea, on the other hand, results from the collapsing of the soft palate and tissues at the back of the throat while one is sleeping, thereby blocking the flow of air. This latter type of sleep apnea is the one most commonly associated with snoring.

Not everyone who snores has sleep apnea. However, if your partner not only snores noisily, but also seems to stop breathing intermittently, then evaluation might be in order. This condition is often seen in people who are obese, although the relationship to the obesity is uncertain.

To receive an objective diagnosis, it's necessary to check into a hospital sleep lab. Sleep specialists hook the patient up to a brain wave monitor, a breathing monitor, and a heart rate monitor, as well as a device to measure the oxygen in the blood. By watching the breathing pattern while the patient sleeps overnight in the hospital, the sleep specialists can determine the presence and type of sleep apnea.

Once sleep apnea is diagnosed, various forms of therapy are possible. Weight loss is the first line of treatment to be considered. If this doesn't work, then something called CPAP (continuous positive airway pressure) is useful. This is a small mask that fits over the nose and creates a continuous flow of airway pressure during sleep in order to prevent the soft tissues of the mouth and palate from collapsing, thereby allowing a free flow of air. In addition, surgery can be performed on the tissues toward the back of the mouth to "tighten them up" which helps to reduce the obstruction. Sleeping on one's side, as opposed to one's back, is also useful as it lessens the gravity effect that contributes to the collapse of the soft tissues.

As a result of many studies, physicians are now aware of a variety of causes of sleep disorders. In fact, it's becoming a new specialty. If you have excessive daytime drowsiness and/or excessive snoring with stoppage of breathing, talk to your doctor about a sleep lab study.

SMOKING

10 WAYS TO SAY GOOD-BYE TO A BAD HABIT

Smoking reduces the oxygen content and increases the carbon monoxide in your bloodstream. If that isn't bad enough, it also causes cancer of the lungs and heart attacks. It is even associated with cancer of the mouth. If cold facts alone aren't persuasive enough, here are some suggestions that might help you quit smoking. Keep in mind that smoking is both a physical and psychological addiction, so you will be tackling two problems at the same time.

- Although "cold turkey" is the best method, cutting back to one cigarette after each meal and at bedtime can help you to taper off gradually and ultimately quit.
- Behavior modification might help. Write down when you smoke each cigarette and describe your activities and feelings at the time. Try to change your behavior pattern and your routine. Avoid those situations that seem to trigger the need for a cigarette.
- Don't go to bars, restaurants, and other places where you usually smoke and where there are lots of other smokers.

- A gum that contains nicotine, if the directions are followed correctly, can help you quit in six to eight weeks.
- Avoid caffeine and other stimulants; these just seem to increase the need for a cigarette.
- Chew celery, carrots, sugar-free gum.
- Put a pack of cigarettes in a jar of water and leave it around the house. When you get the urge to smoke, open up the jar and take a whiff!
- Consider hypnosis, but choose a hypnotist carefully.
- Relaxation techniques help. Listen to soft music and consciously try to breathe deeply and relax when you have the urge to smoke.
- If all else fails, start biting your fingernails or steal your child's pacifier! Anything to help you quit!

SNACK FOODS

WHICH ARE GOOD CHOICES?

Americans love to snack. Unfortunately, many of us don't pay attention to what we are eating or what it contains. Here are the thumbs up and thumbs down for some of the more popular snacks:

- Potato chips are at the bottom of the barrel when it comes to nutrition. They contain some vitamin C, but their outrageous salt content and high caloric value keeps them off our recommended list.
- Peanuts are a poor alternative, even though they're rich in protein and niacin. They simply have too many calories. Even the dry-roasted ones are too fattening. Of course, salt adds to the problem with peanuts.
- Pretzels are an improvement since they're low in calories and fat. Their drawback is that they are made from bleached and unenriched flour and have a high salt content.
- Cheese and crackers aren't bad either. At least they provide some protein and calcium. If you use low-fat cheese and

whole-wheat crackers, you have a pretty good snack.

- The winner in the popular snack category, is popcorn. It's low in calories and high in fiber. Just don't use too much butter or salt.
- If you would like to munch without any guilt at all, you should consider fresh vegetables. A full 60 minutes of crunching on carrots, celery, or other vegetables will give you fewer calories than you would pack away during a single TV commercial using any of the other snacks!

SOFT AEROBICS

A WISER WAY TO EXERCISE

Running is a popular form of hard aerobic exercise. The body must withstand three to four times more impact during running than it does with a softer aerobic exercise like walking. For many people this constant pounding results in damage to the knees and ankles. The bumping and jarring of hard aerobics can cause a breakdown in the body's muscular and skeletal systems. Most of the hard-impact type injuries occur in the legs and feet.

Because of this excessive wear and tear, fitness experts are now recommending a more moderate form of aerobics, thus opening the door to exercise for just about everyone. This is fortunate for those over 40 whose bodies are less likely to withstand the punishment!

Soft aerobic exercise includes swimming, walking, bicycling, and no-impact dance aerobics. These are the same exercises used for rehabilitation by physical therapists. You get a good cardiovascular workout—in fact, about the same as the hard aerobic exercises but without the excessive strain on the joints and muscles.

TO BE MANAGED, NOT ELIMINATED

Stress is an unavoidable part of everyday living. In fact, if we don't feel stress, we're probably not participating in the mainstream of activity. Unfortunately, stress accounts for quite a few medical problems. Headaches, ulcers, high blood pressure, colitis, skin problems, and even heart disease can develop as a result of stress. Although the symptoms and results of stress vary widely, it is important to realize that if they are ignored they will continue to wear down the body and eventually cause damage that can't be reversed.

The best way to manage stress is to first identify its cause. Second, look for more positive ways to interpret stressful events. Our level of stress depends in part on the way we see a problem. The same event happening to two different people can cause one to see it as a threat and another to see it as a marvelous opportunity. Third, learn to anticipate situations that lead to stress. Once you are able to do that, you can plan more effectively for those inevitable changes in your life.

A most useful stress-reducing technique is to allot at least 15 minutes a day for a quiet time by yourself. Simply relax, meditate, or pray. Slow, deep breathing, using your abdomen instead of your chest, can also be very effective.

Remember, while we can't totally eliminate stress from our lives, we can change the way we perceive it, and the way we respond to it.

SUDDEN DEATH IN YOUNG ATHLETES

DON'T EXERCISE WHEN YOU HAVE A VIRUS OR ARE TAKING MEDICATIONS

High school and college competitive sports can be intensely rigorous. For some athletes just recovering from a viral infection, sports can be fatal.

Viruses are the most common cause of a heart infection called myocarditis (inflammation of the heart). This disease can cause the heart to beat irregularly. Depending on the severity of the infection, too much exercise can increase this irregularity to the point where the heart does not pump effectively and can even lead to sudden death. Unfortunately, coaches often are not very sympathetic to a young athlete who has a cold or is on medication. Medications, especially decongestants, can increase the heart's irregularity even further.

Athletes need to be especially careful to listen to their own bodies. If you begin to feel tired and experience body aches from a viral infection, you need to avoid strenuous exercise. If you are having unusual shortness of breath, it is important to stop and rest. Don't overexert yourself, especially if you are on cold medications.

Anyone who still needs medication probably shouldn't be playing. Parents should remember that if a child is beginning to feel better, but still requires some medication, it's best to play it safe and have them avoid strenuous exercise.

SUNSHINE AND SKIN CANCER

RADIATION EXPOSURE ADDS UP

It's a popular misconception that a person who is well tanned is healthy. What that deep brown tan really means is that the skin is putting up a defense against the harmful radiation of the sun. Even the fats in the skin break down as a result of radiation. All this happens on the surface in an attempt to protect the more delicate layers of skin below the surface. The real trouble comes 15 to 20 years later, when premature wrinkling and skin cancer begin to develop.

It is important to limit your exposure to the sun and to use suntan lotion and/or sun screen if you are forced into a situation where you will have high exposure to its harmful rays. The dose of radiation that you begin to get as a child accumulates, and it is this accumulated radiation over many years (15 to 20) that leads to premature wrinkling and skin cancer.

A note about tanning booths: It's easy to get overexposed, and chronic use of tanning booths in search of the "year-round tan" will accelerate the negative effects of the light rays on the skin. Beware of using tanning booths frequently.

THINK HEALTHY—STAY HEALTHY!

A POSITIVE ATTITUDE IS PREVENTIVE MEDI-CINE

Some of us occasionally feel down, in the doldrums, even depressed, and we seem to get sick more often during these times. Did you know many experts feel that your attitude toward life affects your health? It seems people who are more cheerful and who take time to "smell the roses" have fewer problems with sickness. I've seen this in my medical practice. A cheerful outlook won't prevent the development of all disease states, but it can make treatment easier and sometimes more effective. An amazing transformation takes place in people who become very sick, perhaps to the point of near-death, and then get well again. Most people who go through that experience suddenly find that their family relationships are more meaningful, the flowers are more beautiful, and life is more precious. It seems that the worse the illness, the more spectacular the change in attitude, and the greater the meaning of life becomes.

My advice is to try to improve your outlook now in order to avoid getting sick. Don't be one of those people who has to get sick in order to get well!

THORACIC OUTLET SYNDROME

A LITTLE KNOWN CAUSE OF CHEST PAIN AND NUMBNESS IN THE HANDS

In the same way that carpal tunnel syndrome can cause numbness and tingling in the hands, a condition called thoracic outlet syndrome can give very similar symptoms of numbness and tingling, not only in the hand and lower arm, but also in the upper arm, shoulder, neck, and collarbone area.

There is a unique anatomy of the blood vessels and nerves as they come out of the neck and progress toward the arm. It is possible for an abnormal muscle in the neck area, an extra rib, or even some scar tissue from a previous accident to press on these blood vessels and nerves and cause symptoms of pain and numbness in the upper chest, neck, and down the arm. When this is mistaken for heart disease it can be frightening.

This pressure on the blood vessels and nerves accompanies certain motions and positions such as overhead arm exertion, reading the paper, and driving.

People with the most prominent symptoms usually have an extra rib coming off the lower neck vertebrae. However, these symptoms can be caused by conditions other than thoracic outlet (for example, spinal disc injury or arthritis in the neck).

If you have persistent shoulder and arm pain that can't seem to be diagnosed or treated, ask you doctor to consider checking you for thoracic outlet syndrome. Special exercises can relieve the symptoms. Occasionally, surgery might be necessary to remove the extra rib or to split the muscles.

REMOVE THEM PROMPTLY TO AVOID INFECTION

Dad, mom, the kids, the dog — doesn't everyone enjoy a country outing in nice weather? Don't forget to check for ticks — those pesky hitchhikers are out there in grassy and wooded areas just waiting to catch a ride home on you.

Ticks are basically dirty creatures. They carry all sorts of bacteria. Not all of them are serious to humans, but significant diseases like Rocky Mountain spotted fever, tick fever, and Lyme disease are all produced by infectious agents carried by ticks.

A tick first attaches to the skin and then begins to excavate a hole in the skin. Meanwhile, it secretes a cement that firmly binds it to the host. This cement actually causes some of the itchiness of the tick bite. It is important to remove ticks as quickly as possible in order to reduce the opportunity for disease transmission.

Popular remedies for removal have included applying petroleum jelly, fingernail polish, or alcohol to the tick, or touching it with a hot kitchen match (after the flame has been extinguished, of course). But the best method is simply to remove the tick forcibly with the following technique:

1. Use a blunt curved forceps or tweezers to remove the tick. Don't handle the tick with your bare hands because the infectious agents can enter through the skin. Shield your fingers with rubber gloves, a tissue, or a paper towel so you don't have to touch the tick directly.

2. Grasp the tick as close to the skin surface as possible and pull upward with a steady, even pressure. Don't twist or jerk; you don't want the head and mouth parts to break off. Don't squeeze, crush or puncture the body of the tick, because doing so can release the saliva, which is usually where the germs are located.

3. After removing the tick, thoroughly disinfect the bite area with alcohol and wash your hands with soap and water.

It is important to check your children for ticks after they have been out in a wooded area. Ticks often attach themselves near the hairline on the back of the head. If no ticks are found but your children come down with a mysterious illness including fever, aching muscles, headaches, severe pain around the eyes, and perhaps a rash, make sure you see your doctor as soon as possible. Although some of these tick diseases can be fatal, with prompt treatment they can also be cured.

TINNITUS

IT'S NOT MUSIC TO THE EARS

There's an annoying ringing in the ears of nearly 36 million Americans. It disturbs them during the day and keeps them up at night. The noise level can vary from a low roar to a very high-pitched squeal. Tinnitus, as it's called, can occur in one or both ears and be either intermittent or continuous. Some people are so severely afflicted that they cannot lead normal lives.

Most causes of this ailment are not serious. An abnormality of the hearing nerve, often stemming from overexposure to loud noises, or the aging process itself are probably the most common causes of tinnitus. Some feel that abnormalities of the circulation are responsible. Often, however, there is no identifiable cause for this bothersome problem.

There are several measures that might help you find relief from tinnitus:

- Get adequate rest.
- Avoid caffeine and nicotine.
- Decrease salt intake.
- Exercise daily.
- Explore the applications of biofeedback (relaxation and concentration exercises).

Tinnitus is usually more bothersome when you are in a quiet room. A competing sound, such as a ticking clock or a radio on low volume, might help to mask the noises in the head. Some people get relief from a small electronic instrument built into an over-the-ear hearing aid which generates a competitive but pleasant sound that masks the tinnitus.

If you suffer from tinnitus, it is important to have a thorough ear examination to rule out hearing loss or other problems.

CLICKING JAW CAN BE BOTH ANNOYING AND PAINFUL

Do you ever have difficulty fully opening your mouth, or does your jaw pop or click when you open or close it? Does it sometimes get stuck or stay locked in the open position?

If so, you probably have temporal mandibular joint disorder (TMJ). This joint, located on either side of the face, is a ball-and-socket joint that permits the mouth to open and close. The problem can be with the joint itself or with the muscles that move it. Symptoms of pain, headache, ringing in the ears, and even hearing loss can also be associated with this ailment.

The most common cause of TMJ is muscle spasm resulting from stress or tension. The TMJ sufferer tends to clench or grind the teeth, leading to more pain and more spasm. Abnormal occlusion of the teeth (improper bite) also causes TMJ problems. So do arthritis of the jaw, trauma to the area, or yawning for prolonged periods with the mouth open too wide.

The treatment varies according to the cause. Moist heat applied to the face with hot, damp washcloths can help the muscle spasm. Muscle relaxants or anti-inflammatory agents or even anti-anxiety agents can be used. Your dentist can make a specially fitted mouthpiece that redistributes the stress on the muscles to eliminate some of the harmful effects of clenching or grinding of the teeth. If malocclusion is the problem, orthodontic treatment might be necessary. More difficult cases might call for surgical intervention.

To help prevent TMJ problems, limit your eating of caramels and other hard-to-chew foods. Be careful not to yawn too wide. Not all persons with malocclusion or clicking joints have TJM problems, but if you think this is the cause, ask your dentist or physician to check it out.

TRAVELER'S DIARRHEA

TIPS TO PREVENT A RUINED VACATION

Getting diarrhea on a trip takes the pleasure out of your vacation. Traveler's diarrhea can be a problem whether you're heading to New York or Mexico. You don't necessarily have to cross any national borders; just going to another state, where the water is somewhat different from home, can cause the problem.

One of the simplest ways to help prevent this problem is to carry some Pepto-Bismol® liquid. This can be bought over the counter and is shown to prevent or decrease the severity of diarrhea in travelers. It is usually taken as 2 tablespoons four times a day. Two Pepto-Bismol® tablets might also be effective, although the liquid seems to work better. Exactly why or how this works nobody is sure. Apparently, the bismuth coats the lining of the intestines and blocks the effects of the toxin secreted by the germs involved. Remember that there is some salicylate or aspirin-type component to this medication, so if you are taking aspirin already there could be a problem with overdosage. In addition, it might make your stools turn dark or even black, which could mimic bleeding.

Using antibiotics to *prevent* traveler's diarrhea has been a subject of considerable debate. At this time, most experts feel that the risks probably outweigh the benefits.

There are some antibiotics that, if taken on a daily basis, seem to prevent diarrhea. But serious skin reactions in the form of severe sun sensitivity can occur. Most physicians prefer not to prescribe drugs on a preventive basis, but to wait and treat promptly when the symptoms occur. Some of the newer quinolone drugs (Cipro®), which are also used for urinary tract infections, appear to be effective both in prevention and treatment. Use them only on the advice of your doctor.

Many travelers carry antidiarrhea-type medications in the form of Lomotil® or Imodium® in order to reduce the frequency of diarrhea. However, there are some precautions in using them. First, never take them to prevent diarrhea. Second, do not take them on continuous basis. Third, it is important to follow package instructions carefully, since improper use can cause rupture of the colon. Some experts feel it is better to have the diarrhea occur and get rid of the infection that's inside, rather than to prevent it. Ask your doctor about this.

If you are traveling, have a discussion with your doctor before you go. Find out what he or she recommends for you, based on your age, health, and any current medications that you are taking.

VITAMIN C

WILL IT STOP A COLD IN ITS TRACKS?

Vitamin C is a frequent topic in both the medical and lay press. That's because there are both pros and cons to its use. Some of the side effects of taking too much vitamin C include kidney stones and diarrhea. It can also interfere with the laboratory detection of blood in the urine or stool. If you are having that particular test as part of a physical examination, you should stop taking vitamin C for at least 24 hours before the test.

The literature suggests that the benefits of vitamin C outweigh the disadvantages. Even though vitamin C will not prevent colds completely, it does seem to reduce the length and severity.

Some of the more unusual claims make for vitamin C are that it reduces stress, controls cancer pain, and even prevents some forms of cancer. These claims have not been proved.

Various authorities suggest taking anywhere from 500 to 10,000 mg per day. I favor a more conservative course of 500 to 1000 mg per day and then increasing that dose, perhaps up to 3,000 to 5,000 mg, at the onset of a cold.

If you take large doses (more than 5,000 mg) of vitamin C daily, avoid stopping it suddenly. Vitamin C is used to prevent scurvy, and sudden cessation can lead to "rebound scurvy."

THE WEIGHT YO-YO

THE LOSE-GAIN WEIGHT CYCLE: IS IT RISKY?

Many dieters lose and gain hundreds of pounds in a lifetime. Is it unhealthy to lose and then regain weight many times over? The answer is yes, this yo-yo weight fluctuation is unhealthy. There is evidence that when a significant amount of weight is lost, say 10 pounds or more, and then regained, hardening of the arteries is encouraged by the sudden increase in blood fats released into the circulation.

Diminishing muscle tissue is another negative effect of repeated weight loss, especially if the weight is lost through aggressive dieting rather than exercise. Much of the weight that is lost initially is in the form of muscle tissue rather than fat. When the weight is regained, however, it comes back in the form of fat! This seesaw pattern of weight loss and gain is one that ultimately trades what you do want (muscle) for what you don't want (flab)! In addition, many severe diets do not include all of the vitamins and nutrients essential to your health.

The best way to lose weight and keep it off is to do it slowly—not more than 2 pounds per week. Reduce the calories that you get from fats, sugars, and alcohol. And increase your physical activity so you don't tear down your muscles while trying to lose weight.

THE FOLLOWING LAY MEDICAL INFORMATION MAY BE USEFUL:

• DCI Publishing — P.O.Box 47945, Minneapolis, MN 55447-9727. Numerous books on lay medical topics. Send for catalogue.

• *Executive Fitness Newsletter* — Rodale Press, Inc., 33 E. Minor St., Emmaus, PA 18098; $30 per year

• *Harvard Health Letter* — Harvard Medical School Health Publication Group, 164 Longwood Ave., Boston MA 02115 ; $24 per year

• *Health Gazette* — P.O.Box 1786, Indianapolis, IN 46206; $19.95 per year

• *Mayo Clinic Health Letter* — Mayo Foundation for Medical Education and Research, 200 First St. SW, Rochester, MN 55905; $24 per year

• *Medical Update* — P.O. Box 10902, Des Moines, IA 50340

Index

Acetaminophen, 6, 22, 36, 41
Adrenaline kits, 2, 8
AIDS, 52
Alcohol
    and arthritis, 40
    and blood pressure, 12, 53
    and depression, 15
    and hangovers, 41
    and headaches, 44
    and insomnia, 55
    limiting, 51
    and motion sickness, 66
Allergies, 2, 8-9, 30, 42-43, 72
American Cancer Society, 61
American Heart Association, 12
Analgesics, 22
Angina, 46-47
Antihistamines, 2, 19, 22, 26, 43, 56
Antitussives, 22, 23
Appendicitis, 24
Arteries, 10,11
Arthritis, 24, 31, 40, 72
Aspirin, 6, 22, 36, 41, 72
Attitude, 87-88

Bad breath, 40-41
Bleeding, 5
Blindness, 28, 39
Blood clots, 1
Blood sugar, 14, 28, 29
Bronchodilator, 2

Caffeine, 3, 55, 71, 90
Calcium, 70
Cancer, 18, 19, 24-25
    of the breast, 61, 70
    and fiber, 37
    of the lungs, 82
    of the prostate, 73
    of the skin, 86-87
    and vitamin C, 94

Carbon monoxide, 19, 45
Cardiac problems, 17, 34, 36
Chewing gum, 45
Chicken pox, 6
Choking, 27
Cholesterol, 4, 5, 20, 24
        and eggs, 32-33
        and fiber, 37
        and heart attack, 46, 69, 80
Crohn's disease, 23, 24
Cigarettes, 19
Circulation, 1, 20, 68
Colds, 1, 93-94
Colitis, 23, 56, 57
Coma, 6
Constipation, 56
Continuous positive airway pressure, 81-82
Cortisone, 9, 16, 43, 73

Decongestants, 22, 26, 86
Diarrhea, 24, 56, 68, 92-93
Diastolic blood pressure, 10,11
Diet
        and eggs, 32
        and fiber, 37-38
        and longevity, 59
        and obesity, 35
        and snacks, 83-84
        and type II diabetes, 29
        and weight loss, 94
Dietary fiber, 4, 25, 37-38, 57
Diverticular disease, 37
DPT vaccine, 54

Ears, 1, 32, 90-91
Electrocardiogram, 79
Epstein-Barr (EB) virus, 65-66
Exercise
        aerobic, 84
        and back pain, 6
        and blood pressure, 12, 53
        and injury, 76-77
        and headaches, 45
        and heart attacks, 69

Sphygmomanometer, 11
Spike heels, 45
Spinal tap, 64
Strep throat, 75, 76
Stress, 44, 57, 71, 85, 94
Stroke, 9, 11, 12, 28, 46
Sun, 45
Systolic blood pressure, 10, 11

Tear production, 9-10
Teeth, 4
Tick fever, 89
Tylenol. See Acetaminophen

Ulcerative colitis, 23
Ulcers, 3

Viruses, 18-19, 21, 36, 63-64, 65-66, 86
Vitamin A, 4, 31, 62
Vitamin B, 31, 62
Vitamin C, 3, 4, 21, 31, 62, 93-94
Vitamin D, 63, 70
Vitamin E, 31, 63
Vomiting, 6, 44, 47, 63, 68

Weight loss
        and blood pressure, 12
        and colitis, 24
        and diet, 94
        and obesity, 35
        and type II diabetes, 28, 29

Notes

Notes

Notes

CHRONIMED/DCI Publishing Books of Related Interest

When You're Sick and Don't Know Why: Coping with Your Undiagnosed Illness by Linda Hanner, John J. Witek, M.D., with Robert B. Clift, Ph.D. This warm and comprehensive guide offers hope and practical advice for dealing with an undiagnosed illness and for obtaining an accurate diagnosis as quickly as possible.
"Reassuring, helpful, and broadly applicable" — Mary Hager, *Newsweek*.
004087, ISBN 0-937721-83-2, $9.95

Diagnosing Your Doctor by Arthur R. Pell, Ph.D. Authoratative, straightforward, and powerful, this book tells how to get the most from doctors and medical professionals — and shows you how to ask tough questions to get the right answers.
004090, ISBN 0-937721-87-5, $9.95

Minute Health Tips: Medical Advice and Facts at a Glance by Thomas Welch, M.D. This valuable and easy-to-use guide discusses routine health problems, offers preventive medicine tips, shows you how to make doctor visits more informational, and much more.
004088, ISBN 0-937721-85-9, $8.95

Doctor, Why Do I Hurt So Much? by Mark H. Greenberg, M.D., and Lucille Frank, M.D. In clear language and with the latest medical information, two highly renowned rheumatologists show how to combat your arthritis-like condition and start enjoying an active life.
004091, ISBN 0-937721-88-3, $11.95

Emergency Medical Treatment: Infants — A Handbook of What to Do in an Emergency to Keep an Infant Alive Until Help Arrives by Stephen Vogel, M.D., and David Manhoff, produced in cooperation with the National Safety Council. This easy-to-follow, step-by-step guide tells exactly what to do during the most common, life-threatening situations you might encounter for infants. Fully illustrated and indexed with thumb tabs.
004582, ISBN 0-916363-01-5, $7.95

Emergency Medical Treatment: Children — A Handbook of What to Do in an Emergency to Keep a Child Alive Until Help Arrives by Stephen Vogel, M.D., and David Manhoff, produced in cooperation with the National Safety Council. This easy-to-follow, step-by-step guide tells exactly what to do during the most common, life-threatening situations you might encounter for children. Fully illustrated and indexed with thumb tabs.
004583, ISBN 0-916363-00-7, $7.95

Emergency Medical Treatment: Adults — A Handbook of What to Do in an Emergency to Keep an Adult Alive Until Help Arrives by Stephen Vogel, M.D., and David Manhoff, produced in cooperation with the National Safety Council. This easy-to-follow, step-by-step guide tells exactly what to do during the most common, life-threatening situations you might encounter for adults. Fully illustrated and indexed with thumb tabs.
004584, ISBN 0-916363-05-8, $7.95

The Physician Within by Catherine Feste. Here, internationally renowned health motivation specialist, Cathy Feste, focuses on motivating those with a heatlh challenge, and anyone else, to stay on their regimen and follow healthy behavior..

004019,   ISBN 0-937721-19-0, $8.95

Whole Parent/ Whole Child: A Parent's Guide to Raising a Child with a Chronic Illness by Patricia Moynihan, R.N. P.N.P., M.P.H., and Broatch Haig, R.D., C.D.E.   Everything parents of children with chronic health conditions need to know is here. With authority, insight, and compassion, this book shows you how to be the kind of parent you want to be and how to help your child lead the fullest life possible..

004051,   ISBN 0-937721-53-0, $9.95

I Can Cope: Staying Healthy with Cancer by Judi Johnson, R.N., Ph.D., and Linda Klein. This book is a clear, comprehensive resource for anyone whose life has been touched by cancer.   And it's by Judi Johnson, co-founder of the American Cancer Society's internationally acclaimed "I Can Cope" program, which helps over 40,000 people a year.

004026,   ISBN 0-937721-28-X, $8.95

Making the Most of Medicare: A Personal Guide Through the Medicare Maze by Arthur R. Pell, Ph.D.   Finally, a book that actually helps overcome the goverment red tape associated with Medicare.   It shows what can and cannot be expected from Medicare and provides easily understood explanations of Medicare policies — plus tips on how to use them for optimum advantage.

004071,   ISBN 0-937721-66-2, $11.95

Retirement: New Beginnings, New Challenges, New Successes by Leo Hauser and Vincent Miller. From two internationally renowned motivational speakers, trainers and retirees comes a book that will help you achieve new goals in retirement.   It's a plan of action that charts a course to successful, rewarding, and active retirement

004059,   ISBN 0-937721-59-X, $5.95

Fast Food Facts by Marion Franz, RD. This revised and up-to-date best-seller shows how to make smart nutritional choices at fast food restaurants—and tells what to avoid.   Includes complete nutrition information on more than 1,000 menu offerings from the 32 largest fast food chains.

Standard-size edition   004068,   ISBN 0-937721-67-0, $6.95
Pocket edition   004073,   ISBN 0-937721-69-7, $4.95

Convenience Food Facts by Marion Franz, RD, MS, and Arlene Monk, RD. Includes complete nutrition information, tips, and exchange values on over 1,500 popular name-brand processed foods commonly found in grocery store freezers and shelves.   It helps you plan easy-to-prepare, nutritious meals.

004081,   ISBN 0-937721-77-8, $9.95